ASHTANGA YOGA

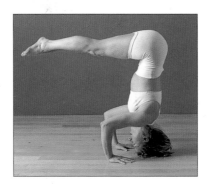

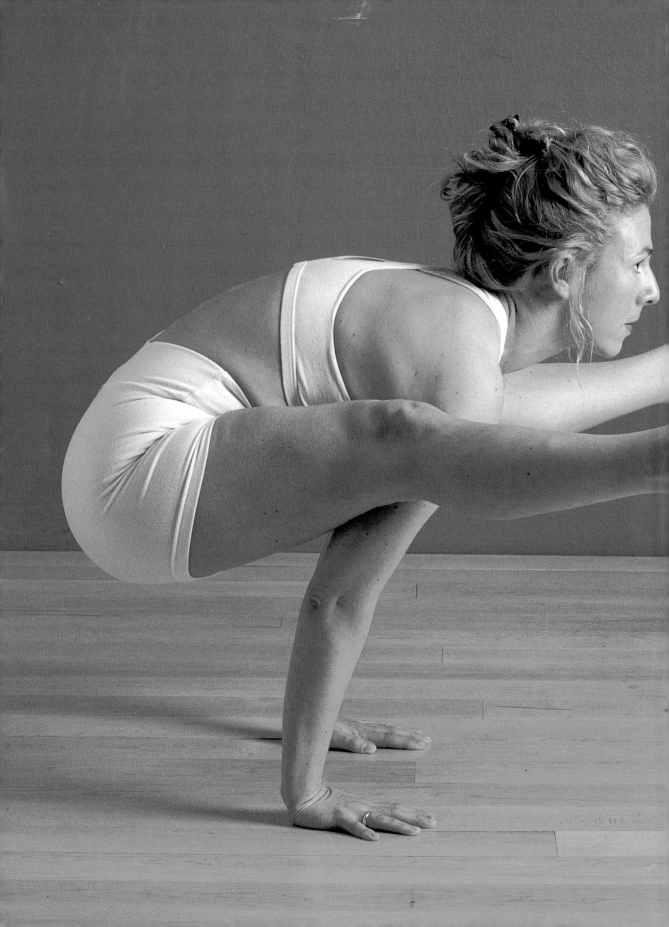

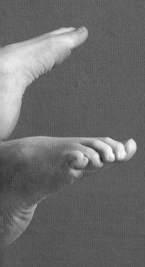

ASHTANGA YOGA

John Scott

Gaia Books Limited

A GAIA ORIGINAL

Books from Gaia celebrate the vision of Gaia, the self-sustaining living Earth, and seek to help its readers live in greater personal and planetary harmony.

Editor	Jonathan Hilton
Designer	Margaret Sadler
Illustrator	John Scott
Photographers	Paul Forrester and Colin Bowling
Managing Editor	Pip Morgan
Production	Lyn Kirby
Direction	Joss Pearson, Patrick Nugent

® This is a Registered Trade Mark of Gaia Books Limited

First published in the United Kingdom in 2000 by
Gaia Books Ltd, 66 Charlotte Street, London W1P 1LR
and 20 High Street, Stroud, Gloucestershire GL5 1AZ

ISBN 1-85675-181-3

A catalogue record of this book is available from the British Library.

Printed in China

10 9 8 7 6 5 4 3 2 1

CONTENTS

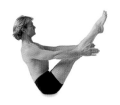

DEDICATION

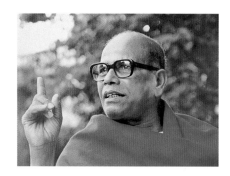

To my beloved and revered Guru, Shri K Pattabhi Jois,
who, with the greatest of love and patience, continues to
show me the way of yoga, I humbly dedicate this work.
It is with the greatest of respect that I attempt to
pass on a little of his teachings to those students who do
not have the good fortune to study directly under his
sensitive and expert tutelage. It is with love and appreciation
that I bow to his lotus feet.

Opening Mantra

Om
Vande Gurunam charanaravinde
Sandarshita svatmasukavabodhe
Nishreyase jangalikayamane
Samsara halahala mohashantyai

Abahu Purushakaram
Shankhacakrsi dharinam
Sahasra sirasam svetam
Pranamami patanjalim
Om

Om
I pray to the lotus feet of the supreme guru
Who teaches knowledge, awakening the great happiness of the
　Self revealed
Who acts like the jungle physician
Able to remove the delusion from the poison of conditioned
　existence

To Patanjali, an incarnation of Adisesa, white in colour with a
　thousand radiant heads (in his form as the divine serpent,
　Ananta), human in form below the shoulders, holding the
　sword of discrimination, a wheel of fire representing infinite
　time, and the conch representing divine sound to him,
I prostrate.
Om

FOREWORD

As the Guru and teacher of John Scott, I am pleased to be able to say a few words to support this book that John has produced in accordance with the traditional method as I have taught it. Ashtanga is a very fine yoga method, having its roots firmly established in the Indian culture since time immemorial. It brings me great joy that the fruits of this yoga system have reached students worldwide. Ashtanga yoga is helping many people throughout the world to balance the mental, physical and spiritual pressures and stresses posed by the modern world we live in today.

Yoga was once regarded as a spiritual practice, suited only to sannyasins or people living an absolute celibate life. This has changed and it has been my duty to my guru, Shri Tirumali Krishnamacharya, to pass on the teachings of this fine method and to share it with as many people as possible, for the greater good. It rewards me to see so many of my fine students continuing to pass on the teachings and subsequent benefits of Ashtanga yoga. The traditional method of teaching is passing down the method directly from guru to student and in this book John refers many times for the need to learn the practice directly from a qualified teacher.

The step by step presentation of this book is a clear and precise representation of the practice method, and can be used to enhance the study of Ashtanga Yoga. I have often said "One percent is theory and ninety-nine percent is practice". It is the 'doing' or the daily practice that brings the many benefits and rewards. John Scott is my good student. He has written this fine book showing the correct method of Ashtanga Yoga. I give my blessing to John, this book and to the students who read it.

Om

Shri K Pattabhi Jois

Introduction

 At the age of 27, after following a conventional career in industrial design, the urge to travel, to leave my home in New Zealand, to discover something more fulfilling to do with my life, lead me in the direction of Greece. Here I found myself on Skiros, at a place called *Atsitsa*, a holistic health and fitness centre, where I worked as a handyman. Funnily enough, my design background was to prove useful in this role – building huts and designing bamboo fixtures and fittings.

Atsitsa offered its residents a variety of activities, including my true passion at the time: windsurfing. In addition, there was dance, paint your dreams, early-morning hum, swimming, tai chi, and yoga. My leisure hours, however, were taken up with windsurfing, the other options being just too "alternative" for me at that time.

During my six months at *Atsitsa* I was fortunate to meet Derek Ireland, a powerfully inspirational man who was responsible for introducing me to Ashtanga Yoga. Derek blasted away all my misconceptions about yoga. The form he showed me was dynamic; its aerobic qualities utilized a unique form of breath technique linked to movement that achieved a graceful, flowing animated sequence. This was utterly different from anything I had ever associated with yoga. Derek is truly responsible for turning me from Commercial Designer to Yoga Student.

In 1989 I travelled to south India to continue my study of yoga with Shri K Pattabhi Jois and his grandson, Sharath, at the Ashtanga Yoga Research Institute, Mysore. I soon came to learn from Shri K Pattabhi Jois, the current guru of Ashtanga Yoga, that this form of yoga is a very ancient system with a long lineage of gurus and its own traditions.

As a 13-year-old youth, Shri K Pattabhi Jois (Guruji) became the student of Shri Krishnamacharya, a renowned Indian guru who is reputed to have lived to be 101. Guruji worked hard and became one of Krishnamacharya's advanced students and, eventually, the beneficiary of the secrets and techniques of yoga Asana and Philosophy (*see pp. 14–17*). Together, Krishnamacharya and Guruji translated an ancient text, *Yoga Korunta*, and refined the system of yoga, known as Ashtanga, that has become increasingly popular throughout the Western world. Today, in his eighties, Guruji continues to teach as many as 70 students a day. He is a remarkable man with boundless energy and I have been fortunate to have

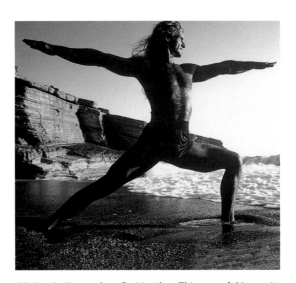

My inspiration and my first teacher. This powerful image is of Derek Ireland, seen in a pose from the Warrior Sequence (Virabhadrasana), on a deserted beach on Crete, Greece.

had so many years of continuing study with him, experiencing the magic and power of his touch.

The feature that truly distinguishes Ashtanga Yoga from the other forms of yoga practised today is its unique movement/breathing system, or *vinyasa*. Movement through the sequence of poses (*asanas*) is responsible for producing heat, which, in turn, produces sweat. The sweat is both cleansing and purifying, initiating the release of toxins retained within the superficial fat layers of the body. As students progress more deeply into the practice, toxins held in the deeper layers of muscle tissue and internal organs are also released, resulting in a healthy, toned, and flexible body.

The Power of the Breath (*see pp. 18–23*) cannot be overestimated, since it is key to this system of yoga. The breath is energizing, calming, and meditative. The breath is called *ujjayi*; its sound, volume, and rhythm are powerful. It draws the mind in on itself and, in so doing, yolks mind and body together. It is the breath, *bandhas*, and *dristis* (the three core techniques of vinyasa – *see pp. 20–3*) that, when applied together, bring about the physical and the meditative aspects of Ashtanga Yoga. The practice itself (once the student is experienced enough to stop thinking about which asana comes next) becomes a moving meditation. But this grace can only become real when all the aspects of the practice come together in harmony.

Ashtanga Yoga's ancient roots are a sign of its potency and effectiveness; it has proved to be one of the fastest-growing health and fitness practices in the world today. Many celebrity figures have put their names to the practice and endorse its benefits. For many of them, Ashtanga Yoga is far more than mere exercise – it is responsible for their stamina, focus, feelings of wellbeing, their toned physical bodies, and peace of mind.

This book has been written with the intention of sharing the practices and passing on the teachings received from Shri K Pattabhi Jois. There have been many texts written in Sanskrit (the ancient classical root language of India) on the subject of yoga, but there are few texts written in English on Ashtanga Yoga. In this book, the use of step-by-step photography with detailed, instructive text makes the material suitable for both beginners and current students who wish to deepen their understanding of the techniques of vinyasa.

About this book

Many years of practice are needed for Ashtanga Yoga students to develop an understanding of the system's true essence. It is impossible in an introductory book such as this to bring fully to light the depth of practice necessary to achieve the union of mind, body, and soul. What can be done, however, and what this book presents, are the key principles and techniques of the method. It takes a combination of dedication, discipline, motivation, and stamina to achieve any lasting benefit. Ashtanga Yoga is a daily practice, one that ultimately becomes a way of life. I hope that this text is an inspiration to you, encouraging you to take your first "Victorious Breath".

If you are a complete novice, it is not advisable to start Ashtanga Yoga using just a book as guidance. Use the contacts provided at the back of the book to find a certified teacher. Before finding a teacher, however, you can start work on *Surya Namaskara A* and *B*, or Sun Salutes A and B (*see pp. 24–7*). Take care to read all the details of the techniques and note that repetition over consecutive days is the traditional method of learning. Add in new postures one at a time at the start of each new practice day, but only when you are ready. Don't rush. Pay particular attention to counting the breath/movements into and out of each posture.

At the beginning, don't worry about what your postures look like – this will only take your mind away from the focus of the breath. What is crucial is understanding that each breath initiates a movement, and that the breath contains the connection to the bandhas – and it is the application of the bandhas that ensures a safe practice. Before attempting the routines in Sequences 1 to 3 you should have the benefit of a certified teacher.

OPPOSITE *The worship of Lord Shiva includes highly philosophical and ascetic orders. To gain* shivata, *"the nature of Shiva", you must remove the bonds that confine the soul, and yoga (meditation) is one of the paths to this goal.*

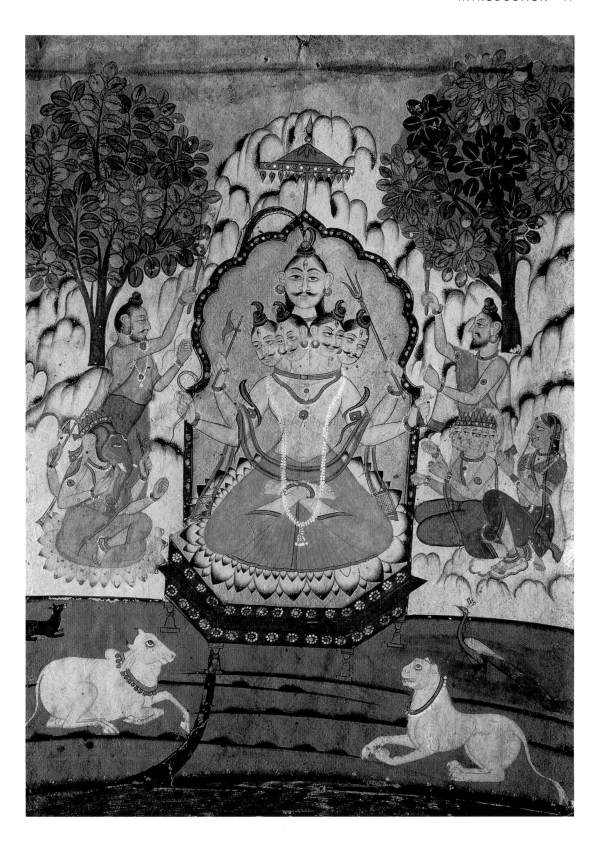

1

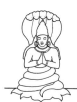

The Way of Ashtanga Yoga

Ashtanga Yoga is a science and a practice that has evolved over a period of thousands of years to deal with moral, physical, mental/emotional, and spiritual development. The term *ashtanga*, which means "eight limbs", was devised in about 200 BC by the great Indian sage Pantanjali. He was the first yogi to systematize an approach to yoga, and his eight-limb system provided then, as it still does today, a set order of steps through which practitioners can progress in order to reach a state of yoga. In this context, "yoga" means the yoking, or union, of mind, body, and soul leading toward self-realization. In order to achieve this union, it is first necessary to take control of the mind and to remove the unnecessary stimuli and clutter that get in the way of clarity. Within the eight-limbed system of Ashtanga, the third limb is *Asana*. This is the practice of classical yoga postures, and it is the device that ties the mind to the body through the "thread of the breath". In this system, the breath becomes the key to the focusing of the mind.

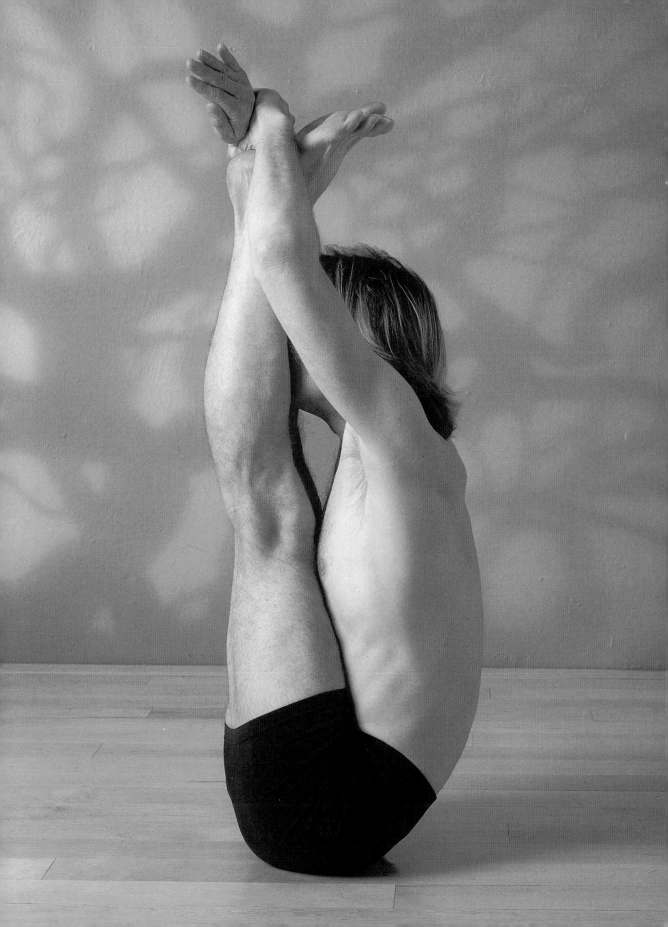

The Eight Limbs of Ashtanga

 In a direct translation from the ancient Sanskrit word *ashtanga*, *ashto* means "eight", while *anga* means "limb" or "stage". The renowned Indian sage Pantanjali, writing more than two thousand years ago, assigns eight limbs to the tree of yoga – each limb being a stage or step along the path to self-realization. In the tradition stemming from this ancient text, each limb of yoga is given in a precise order through which practitioners must progress. Starting from the bottom, these eight stages are: Yama (moral codes); Niyama (self-purification and study); Asana (posture); Pranayama (breath control); Pratyahara (sense control); Dharana (concentration); Dhyana (meditation); and finally Samadhi (contemplation, self-realization, or a state of bliss).

Through his writing, Pantanjali instructs us that all eight stages must be observed and practised in turn in order to purify and yoke (meaning "to unify" in this context) mind, body, and soul. At the end of the journey, the fruits of the tree of yoga are then available to be harvested.

Because the concepts underlying the first two limbs, Yama and Niyama, are initially difficult to grasp for anybody who has not been steeped in Eastern traditions and philosophy since birth, Shri K Pattabhi Jois (Guruji) first introduces his Western students to Asana, the third limb, because it is through the demanding discipline and practice of Asana that students begin to observe and understand the importance of breath control.

PREVIOUS PAGE *When executed with grace, the forward bend radiates qualities of inner peace. This pose appears many times in various guises throughout the practice – balanced, as the one pictured here in* Urdhva Mukha Paschimattanasana; *standing, as in* Surya Namaskara; *or seated. The physical benefits of the forward bend are numerous, but in particular the digestive processes are stimulated and strengthened as a result.*

Through the observance of the ujjayi breath (*see pp. 18–21*), students begin to experience clarity of mind. With this background, students then have some ability to contemplate developing the first and second limbs of yoga.

Yama (moral codes)

Yama comes from the root word *yam*, which means "to restrain". Yama can be divided into five moral codes: Ahimsa (non-violence); Satya (truthfulness); Asteya (non-stealing); Brahmacharya (preserving vital fluids); and Aparigraha (non-possessiveness).

Yama indicates how individuals should respond and to relate to other people and all living beings, and to the environment, in order to achieve a peaceful and harmonious world. In the practice of Asana, students learn that they must first be able to observe all the moral codes in their relationship with themselves in order to relate in the same fashion to the outside world.

Throughout the practice of Asana, students must respect the limits and capabilities of their own bodies. At no point should they force a movement or impose a stretch that causes injury to themselves.

Ahimsa deals with the aspect of non-violent action. When starting the practice of Asana, students will almost certainly become frustrated at some point with the difficulty of achieving a particular posture – the lotus posture, for example, which is the classic meditation pose and requires patience and tolerance to learn. This frustration can cause students to force themselves into the posture without showing due respect for their knees. This will eventually result in injury. These difficult and potentially injurious postures are designed to teach yoga students how to relate to their own bodies, not with violence but with respect and love.

Satya teaches students to be truthful in their relationships with themselves and with others. In the practice of Asana, you need to be honest with yourself and your practice without harbouring egotistical expectations. It is important to accept where your practice is without always striving for more. Practice requires devotion, discipline, and enthusiasm while working within reasonable limits.

Asteya teaches students not to cheat, steal, or be jealous or envious of others. Yoga Asana is a non-competitive practice, and students need to look to their neighbours for inspiration rather than to cast judgements or to make negative comparisons.

Brahmacharya is the discipline designed to prevent practitioners turning to sexual passion at inappropriate times during the month. There are times set down when it is considered appropriate for men and women to enjoy each other's bodies, and although it is unlikely that many people will want to impose what, to Western eyes, appears to be an arbitrary timetable on their sexual activity, the practice of Asana holds to the belief that squandering sexual fluids drains the practitioner's energy and weakens the body.

Aparigraha is concerned with non-possessiveness. In relation to Asana, for example, it is better to practise for the appropriate amount of time neces-sary to maintain your physical health rather than to push yourself too hard because you desire to be better than you are. This part of the moral code of Yama teaches you how to let go of the "attachment to progress" and to allow progress to happen spontaneously. If the demands on you increase for any reason, then allow your practice to reflect your changed circumstances, without you feeling the need to hold on to what you were able to achieve before the change. Sometimes, less is more.

Niyama (self-purification and study)

Ni can be translated as "down" or "into", while *yam* means "to restrain". Niyama can be divided into five codes: Shaucha, Santosha, Tapas, Swad-hyaya, and Ishwarapranidhana, all of which refer to self-cleansing and can be dealt with together.

If Yama is to do with mental purification, then Niyama deals with contentment and physical cleansing – purification of the body – both internally and externally. Spiritual purification is achieved through the recital of Vedic mantras and surrender of the self to God.

Students of yoga address the concepts of Yama and Niyama gradually, certainly over a period of years. Guruji suggests that through the practice of the third limb, Asana, yoga students will begin to regulate their breath and, in so doing, begin to find some clarity of thought. This clarity allows students to relate with kindness, honesty, and respect both to themselves and to others. If these codes are not adhered to, students will not achieve the union of mind and body; instead the postures will act only as another form of exercise, and students will miss the opportunity to harvest the fruit from the tree of yoga.

Asana (posture)

From the word *aas*, meaning "to sit" or "to be", *asana* encompasses the meaning of a particular posture or mode of sitting. "Seat" is the most literal translation of *asana*. Ashtanga Yoga organizes postures (asanas) into three groups. The primary series (Yoga Chikitsa – *see pp. 36–135*) aligns and purifies the body. The intermediate series (Nadi Shodhana) purifies the nervous system. The advanced A, B, C, and D series (Sthira Bhaga) integrates strength with grace of movement. Each series has been precisely arranged and each level must be fully developed before students progress to the next.

The primary series is, therefore, the beginning of Asana practice, and it is within this series that students are introduced to the principles and technique of breath/movement synchronicity (*see pp. 20–3*). This provides the roots and foundation that support the other seven limbs of yoga.

The asana poses have been carefully organized in a specific sequence to access every muscle in the body, stretching and toning them, as well as the nerves, organs, glands, and energy channels. But asanas are not merely exercises; they are postures and transitions synchronized to the breath. It is through *tristana* (the union of vinyasa), *bandhas* (the locks or seals that protect the body), and *dristis* (looking points) that practitioners journey inside, working deeply on the inner body, opening and clearing the *nadis*, the energy channels of the subtle body, allowing themselves to access and harness the internal lifeforce known as *prana*. Only when this pranic energy has been accessed can the yogi transcend the physical body.

By practising asana poses in the prescribed sequence, students gain the necessary stamina, strength, flexibility, and steadiness of mind to sit in *Padmasana*, the classic lotus position (*see pp. 32–3*). Once they can sit in this pose for long periods without discomfort, they can begin practising the fourth and seventh limbs (Pranayama and Dhyana), which take them to higher states of mind than is possible through non-yogic exercise.

Pranayama (breath control)

Prana means "breath", "energy", "strength", or "lifeforce", while *ayama* means "length", "restraint", "expansion", or "stretching". For most of us, breathing is an involuntary reflex action. Yogis, however, appreciate the role breath has in focusing the mind, and Pranayama was developed to control breathing as a method of controlling the mind.

Through the practice of Asana, yoga students slowly begin to learn the dynamics of breath – how to equalize inhalation and exhalation and how to synchronize movement to breath, rather than breath to movement. This requires constant concentration on the flow of breath, and this concentration is the beginning of Pranayama, Pratyahara, and Dharana.

In the early stages of yoga practice, to move into, hold, and then move out of an asana are difficult to achieve, especially while maintaining breath/movement synchronicity and without straining the breath or the body.

Pranayama is an advanced form of control over the inhalation, exhalation, and retention of the breath (holding the breath). You must treat breath control with great respect. Pranayama is a powerful tool, directing energy through the energy channels of the body. In order to work properly and efficiently, these energy channels must be cleaned and cleared and the body made strong through the practice of Asana. The breath, too, must be strong and clear when performing the asana poses before undertaking Pranayama as a separate practice. Students must attain an advanced level of Asana practice before Shri K Pattabhi Jois will instruct them in the art and science of Pranayama.

Pratyahara (sense control)

Prati means "against" or "back", and *haara* means "take hold" – so *Pratyahara* is to "hold back". When you are practising Asana and Pranayama, your mind can easily wander away from concentrating on the inner body to other matters – for example, some imminent social engagement or idle consideration about what is for dinner that evening or suddenly remembering that you need to pick up your trousers from the dry cleaners. Alternatively, your mind can spiral in on a pain in your knee and the pain then becomes the focus.

Pratyahara is the limb of steadiness; it operates by continually bringing the mind back to the rhythm of breath. As a result, the mind is calmed and controlled, and as the focus develops to a higher level students are able to harness and control their senses. When full awareness is achieved, the mind does not waver or latch on to passing thoughts – it simply allows the thought to pass on by. Pratyahara is about sense control. Rather than closing thoughts out, you learn not to become attached to them as they move through your mind. At all times you are fully aware of sensations in your body, and if you have a painful knee, for example, this is acknowledged or supported through releasing the pain using a deliberate, smooth-flowing exhalation.

Dharana (concentration)

The word *dhar* translates as "to hold" or "to maintain". When practitioners achieve a high level of Pratyahara, the mind is undisturbed by stray thoughts, sounds, and sensations, such as pain. In this state, it is possible to achieve a deep level of concentration. Within the practice of Asana, when Dharana is achieved the mind reaches a single focus, concentrating purely on inhalation and exhalation and the looking place, or dristi.

Dhyana (meditation)

Dhyana comes from *dhyai*, which means "to meditate" or "contemplate". The combination of limbs five and six (Pratyahara and Dharana) brings about a state of deep meditation where there is no thought at all. In Asana, the pranic energy of the student flows throughout the sequence of asana postures. From the beginning to the end of the sequence, the thread of the breath is unbroken. Each posture is gracefully strung on a garland of asanas, becoming, in effect, a moving meditation.

Samadhi (contemplation)

Sama means "the same", while *adhi* translates as "the highest". To reach Samadhi is the culmination of all the eight limbs of Ashtanga. It is the goal, the fruit of the tree. To reach this point you have climbed to the very highest reaches of the tree and you can see "all".

It is the fruit that creates the seed for the next generation of trees and it is the fruit that is the edible or ingestibly sweet tasting part of the tree. The fruit is for us to consume, or for us to be consumed within. To reach Samadhi is to become one with God.

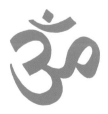

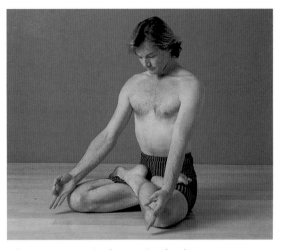

The Lotus posture (Padmasana) is the classic yoga meditation pose. The spine is straight, eyes cast down to the gaze point known as nasagrai, and the focus is drawn inward – to the breath and the bandhas.

The first four limbs of Ashtanga are the external disciplines that, when practised regularly, create the necessary physical and mental state from which the remaining four internal limbs can spontaneously sprout and unfold. Ashtanga Yoga is a tried and tested system. When we seriously apply ourselves to the practice of Asana, combined with ujjayi pranayama and dristi, in such a systematic way, we can begin to liberate the movement of all of the eight limbs of the tree of yoga.

Observing the eight limbs in the practice of Ashtanga Yoga is crucial if you are to taste the fruits of the tree of yoga. Yogi Shri K Pattabhi Jois often says "Do your practice and all is coming". He does not mean that enlightenment will just happen if you practise; he is advising that once the seed has been planted, it has to be tended daily, nurtured, and watered through the discipline of regular practice. As a result of devoted practice, insights sprout from within, and an understanding of the tree of yoga begins to grow. The eight limbs become the tools with which to work the soil. But only if students follow the correct practice method will the tree grow to maturity.

2

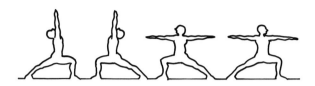

Vinyasa

The essence of the vinyasa element of Ashtanga Yoga is a synchronicity of breath and movement. In vinyasa, the breathing technique called *ujjayi*, or "Victorious Breath", initiates the movement, and then movement and breath flow as one. The characteristic of ujjayi is the soft, sibilant sound made when breathing. Inhalations and exhalations are through the nose; as if drinking the perfume of a rose, the air is taken to the back of the throat where, by a subtle contraction of the muscles around the glottis, its flow is regulated. The quantity and length of inhalations and exhalations are equal, and it is this equality that sets the rhythm and meditative aspects of Ashtanga Yoga. When practising ujjayi, you discover the integral partnership between breath and *bandha*. Meaning "lock" or "seal", each bandha harnesses and directs the pranic qualities of the Victorious Breath. Bandha control requires a fine balance between hard and soft. The correct application will free the breath, unleashing an uplifting effect that imparts internal strength and lightness to the body.

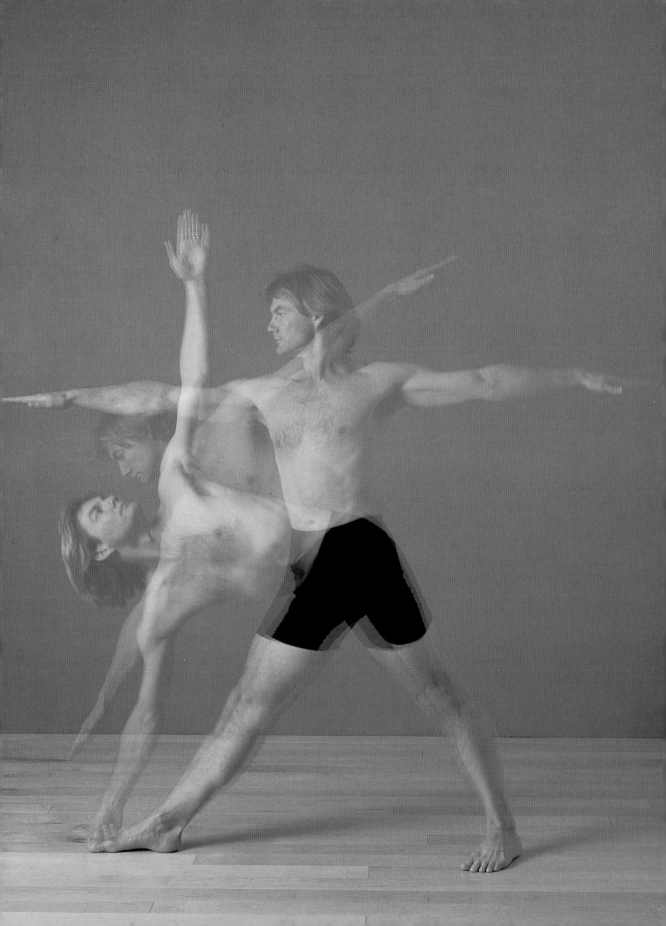

Breath and movement synchronicity
Vinyasa

In a direct translation of the Sanskrit word *vinyasa*, *vi* means "to go", "to move", "to cast forth", "to conceive", or "to start from", while *nyasa* means "placing", "planting", or "prostration". Through their research into the origins of this form of yoga, guru Shri Krishnamacharya (*see p. 9*) and his then student, Shri K Pattabhi Jois, the current guru (Guruji) of Ashtanga Yoga, discovered two important factors. First, all the *asanas*, or "postures", are linked in an exact sequence, and second, there is a precise number of synchronized breath/movement transitions into and out of each asana.

In his book *Yoga Mala*, Shri K Pattabhi Jois details how each asana starts with *Samasthitih* – in which the practitioner stands ready to move with equal breath – and then returns to *Samasthitih*, with an exact number of synchronized breath/movement transitions, or vinyasas, in between.

These principles are introduced right from the beginning with *Surya Namaskara A* (*see pp. 24–5*), in which there are nine counted breath-synchronized movements (vinyasas). For simplicity's sake, the positions are named, but in fact we are counting the transitions from one position to the next in the sequence. Bear in mind that the counting is strictly sequential, so that, say, vinyasa 8 of one sequence may be different to vinyasa 8 of another.

These principles underly the practice of Ashtanga Yoga and are responsible for creating a system that is known for its graceful, flowing sequences of transitions and postures "woven on the thread of the breath". And the three key

PREVIOUS PAGE *This multiexposed image captures something of the dynamic quality of the practice of Ashtanga Yoga – here the second vinyasa of* Utthita Trikonasana *(see pp. 42–3) can be seen.*

components that turn these principles into the actuality of vinyasa are the *ujjayi* (Victorious Breath), the *bandhas*, and the *dristis*. When all three come together, practitioners have reached *tristana*. Having attained tristana, practitioners of Ashtanga Yoga can then begin to practise the sixth and seventh limbs of ashtanga – concentration and meditation (*see pp. 14–17*).

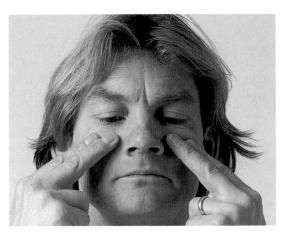

To simulate the dilation of the nostrils, take the first two fingers of each hand and place them on your upper cheeks. Lightly stretch the skin either side of the bridge of your nose to flare the nostrils and breathe at the back of your throat.

Ujjayi

When learning the intricacies of the Victorious Breath, students often find it difficult to produce the correct sound characteristic of ujjayi. To do this, air is drawn in and out through the nose, but the sound should not come from the nostrils. If it does, you are in effect sniffing. When you are moving to the rhythm of the breath, your muscles demand a constant supply of oxygen. To meet this demand, airflow needs to increase – but if you sniff, airflow is, in fact, restricted. To prevent this, each breath is drawn in from the back of the throat so that the airflow can be increased and metered by the muscles around the glottis. It is the friction of air through the glottis that produces the ujjayi sound. This friction also warms the air before it enters the lungs. To help correct any tendency to sniff, lightly stretch the skin either side of the nose to dilate your nostrils (*see left*) so that air is being drawn in at the back of your throat.

The correct ujjayi sound is similar to the noise waves make as they surge up a pebbly beach. To achieve this "free breathing" you must keep the glottis open at all times during the inhalation/exhalation cycle. Closing your glottis is like holding your breath: if this happens, the energy flow stops and your muscles become starved of oxygen and pranic energy, and therefore tighten up. In this state, it could be said that "where there is no breath there is no life", and thus vinyasa and the asana become lifeless.

The grunting noises practitioners sometimes make indicate that the glottis has been locked closed – this usually occurs at the top of the inhalation or at the bottom of the exhalation – and so you need to refocus your attention on keeping the glottis open. This control is the only way to achieve ujjayi. You can practise ujjayi any time you like – when walking, for example, climbing stairs, or even as a part of a relaxation routine.

You can think of the ujjayi technique as the inner stretching of your breath. Once you have mastered this method of controlling the glottis, you next need to turn your attention to metering the length of each breath. There is usually an imbalance between the duration of inhalations and that of exhalations, and so the aim now is to achieve *sama* ("same"), the equalization of both the length and intensity of each inhalation and exhalation.

In the beginning, exhalations are usually longer and easier to achieve. So, the first "stretching of the breath" is to lengthen the inhalation in order to match that of the exhalation. The second stretching of the breath comes when synchronizing breath/movement transitions, when the length of the transition sometimes requires a longer inhalation and/or exhalation. The result of stretching the breath is the stretching of the body.

Bandha

Bandha is the first paradox that we come across in Ashtanga Yoga. *Bandha* means "lock" or "seal", but the result of applying a bandha is to unlock the latent lifeforce energy and then to move and direct this pranic current from its inner source to enter the network of 72,000 *nadi* ("energy channels") of the subtle body. The development of bandha control cultivates and increases prana, and it is from the integration of ujjayi and bandha that an internal alchemy is achieved. When this chemistry is working correctly, the asana is revealed from the inner body, and the outer body eventually reflects that which is created within.

There are three bandhas controlling the sealing of prana: *mula bandha, uddiyana bandha*, and *jalandhara bandha*. All three bandhas are integral components of the ujjayi breathing technique.

Mula bandha This bandha is the root lock or root foundation. It is discovered at the end of the exhalation, when you are "on empty", but it is applied throughout the whole breath cycle. At the end of a complete exhalation, if you are in tune with the natural workings of your body, you will feel a slight sensation as the anal sphincter muscles subtly contract, drawing the entire genital region, including the perineum, inward and upward. This lifting action of what is known as the "pelvic floor" is responsible for the inner muscular support of the lower digestive organs.

Mula bandha is responsible for the root energy necessary for a firm foundation, whether this foundation is the feet, hands, or bottom. Mula bandha is also the safety lock protecting the body, sealing prana internally for the uddiyana bandha then to direct it upward through the nadis.

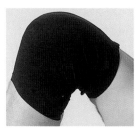 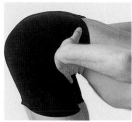

Uddiyana bandha is best practised in the Downward-facing Dog position. During the five breaths taken in this position, practise fully exhaling without tensing your lower abdomen. On the inhalation, try to direct your breath into your back and chest without losing the softness and stillness of your lower abdomen.

The application of uddiyana bandha is shown here on the transition out of a Standing Forward Bend (see p. 39). This pose is bandha-locating. Place your hands on your lower abdomen to check if the application is correct. This bandha helps to protect your lower back when coming out of a forward bend.

Mula bandha is difficult to master. At first it is a gross, general action of squeezing the outer and inner sphincters of the anus. From discovering this gross action, the application of mula bandha becomes lighter, increasingly sensitive – more a subtle lifting of the perineum. The location of the bandha can be experienced differently for men and women, but you can practise it anywhere and at anytime until you get the action just right.

Uddiyana bandha This is the most dynamic of all the bandhas and can be translated as "upward flying". You will most easily discover the position of this bandha at the end of an exhalation – "on empty". This "empty" can best be experienced in the *Adho Mukha Svannasana* (Downward-facing Dog position) of *Surya Namaskara A* (*see above left and pp. 24–5*). This position is held for the duration of five breaths. After six moving transitions to reach this point, you now hold your body stationary to regulate and equalize the rhythm of your breath. It is here that it is best to cultivate the uddiyana and mula bandhas.

Because uddiyana bandha relates directly to the workings of the diaphragm, ribs, and intercostal muscles, it plays a crucially important role in the development of ujjayi breath. During exhalation, the diaphragm relaxes, moving up into the lungs to push the air out, and the internal intercostal muscles pull down the ribcage to complete the action. The result of this is to draw in the abdominal wall (the region from the navel down to the pubis), which supports and protects all the internal organs and the lower back. If your lower abdominal wall is well toned, you can hold the lower abdomen in this position with minimal effort for the entire inhalation/exhalation cycle.

This abdominal control provides a platform, or foundation, for the next incoming breath. As the diaphragm flexes in a downward direction, drawing ujjayi breath into the lungs, the external intercostal muscles lift the ribcage, expanding the thoracic region and allowing the lungs to inflate to their maximum capacity. This is the physical action of uddiyana bandha, which, when perfected, is also a subtle control that results in a "softness and stillness" of the lower abdomen.

To feel the uddiyana bandha in action, it is useful to look at the vinyasa transition out of *Padangusthasana* (Standing Forward Bend – *see above right and pp. 38–9*). This vinyasa is stationary and intended purely for the cultivation of uddiyana bandha and the protection of the lower back. As you can see above, you place your hands on your lower abdomen to connect physically with the bandha. Placing your hands on uddiyana bandha is a frequent action during the standing asanas – it not only reminds you of the function of the bandha, it also provides you with many chances to practise and develop this control.

The paradox of bandha is that the lock in fact unlocks the flowing pranic energy and directs it upward. Uddiyana bandha combined with mula bandha are responsible for the lightness and strength evident in Ashtanga Yoga. The Jump

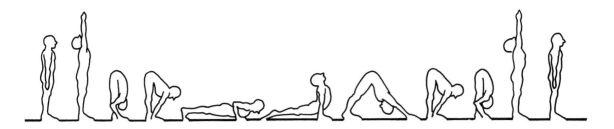

Through vinyasa (*see pp. 70–1*) demonstrates the rooting of mula bandha through the hands and the flight of uddiyana bandha as the legs are floated through the space between the arms – all on a cushion of ujjayi breath.

Uddiyana bandha is a generally beneficial technique, one you can practise during the day. It helps to support your lower digestive organs and to protect the lower back when bending or lifting.

Jalandhara bandha The next bandha, or lock, is jalandhara bandha. This is the third bandha and it occurs spontaneously in a subtle form in many asanas due to the *dristi* ("gaze point"), or head position. Once again, *Surya Namaskara A* (the sixth position) best demonstrates this bandha, as the chin tucks in toward the notch between the collar bones in order to look at the correct dristi – the navel. Primarily, it is a lock specific to *Pranayama*, or "breath control" – the fourth limb of Ashtanga (*see pp. 14–17*). This lock prevents pranic energy escaping and stops any build-up of pressure in the head when holding the breath. It is best to practise jalandhara bandha only under the supervision of an advanced teacher.

Dristi

Each asana in the Ashtanga Yoga system has a gaze point on which to focus. There are nine dristis and each is intended to draw the outward-looking eyes inward. They are, in the order of appearance:
◆ Nasagrai (the tip of the nose)
◆ Angusta ma dyai (the thumbs)
◆ Broomadhya (the third eye)
◆ Nabi chakra (the navel)

This illustration represents the flowing, unbroken wave energy of the Surya Namaskara A. It shows the vinyasas woven on the "thread of breath" – a continuous pulse that can be likened to the rhythm of a heartbeat.

◆ Urdhva (up to the sky)
◆ Hastagrai (the hand)
◆ Padhayoragrai (the toes)
◆ Parsva (the far left)
◆ Parsva (the far right)
Using the discipline imposed by the dristis, the mind becomes focused, taking students "inside". This inner focus leads to the development of concentration (*Dharana*) and meditation (*Dhyana*) – the sixth and seventh limbs of Ashtanga.

Tristana

The true essence of vinyasa is experienced when a state of tristana is achieved. This is the union of the three main focuses of Ashtanga Yoga: advanced breath/movement synchronicity, bandhas, and dristis. When this union blossoms, a powerful wave of fluidity and grace flows out from the practice, and the resulting chemistry unleashes the energies of the five elements:
◆ Earth – mula bandha producing foundation, stability, and strength.
◆ Water – the fluidity of vinyasa producing sweat.
◆ Air – ujjayi breathing and bandhas for lightness.
◆ Fire – the purifying digestive fire of agni.
◆ Ether – the subtle, all-pervading prana.

Tristana is achieved through repetition. It is repetition that brings about the familiarity necessary to make the transitions and postures subtle, natural, and graceful.

Sun Salute A
Surya Namaskara A

Surya Namaskara is the ritual salute to the sun god. When it is practised correctly, it can result in physical and mental health, thus paving the way for spiritual awareness in all aspects of life. Without this central devotional element, yoga would become simply a series of physical exercises.

Surya Namaskara introduces the method that we practise in order to achieve the state called "yoga". This is, in essence, the union of body, mind, and soul, leading eventually to self-realization. The method is *vinyasa*, or breath/movement synchronicity, incorporating the concept of *ujjayi*, or Victorious Breath, which is the rhythmical and equal length of inhalations and exhalations. Integral to the practice of Ashtanga Yoga are the *dristis*, or specific gaze points, and the *bandhas*, or energy seals or locks that channel and direct the flow of internal energy and protect the body. When these three principal techniques merge as one focus, *tristana* (*see p. 23*) is achieved.

Vinyasa literally means "movement/breathing" system – one breath, one synchronized movement. *Surya Namaskara A* has nine vinyasas, which means there are nine movements synchronized to the rhythm of the ujjayi breath, each with its own gaze point. Traditionally, students are counted through the nine vinyasas, thereby setting a continuous rhythm of breath, and the repetition of the nine vinyasas (without stopping or taking extra breaths) introduces the meditative quality to the practice.

Practising dristi and listening to the sound of ujjayi help to draw your focus inside to the breath–bandha connection, and this principle can be explored in the 6th vinyasa, Downward-facing Dog, which is held for five full breaths.

Stemming from the controlled state of mind produced by the repetition of the nine vinyasas, there is also a physical reaction: the body begins to produce an inner heat, and it is this heat that is essential to the process of purification. In addition, it acts to warm the joints and muscles, preparing them for the physical work to follow.

Surya Namaskara A is repeated five times.
Samasthitih: Exhaling, stand in this neutral position, look to your nose.
1 **Ekam:** Inhaling, reach up, look up to your thumbs.
2 **Dve:** Exhaling, forward bend, look to your nose.
3 **Trini:** Inhaling, lift your head, look to your third eye.
4 **Chatvari:** Exhaling, jump back, look to your nose.
5 **Panca:** Inhaling, roll to Upward-facing Dog, look to your third eye.
6 **Shat:** Exhaling, roll to Downward-facing Dog, look to your navel (5 breaths).
7 **Sapta:** Inhaling, jump up, look to your third eye.
8 **Ashtau:** Exhaling, forward bend, look to your nose.
9 **Nava:** Inhaling, reach up, look to your thumbs.
Samasthitih: Exhaling, return to this neutral position, look to your nose.

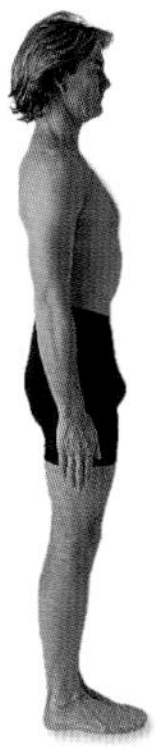

▲ Samasthitih
Exhale

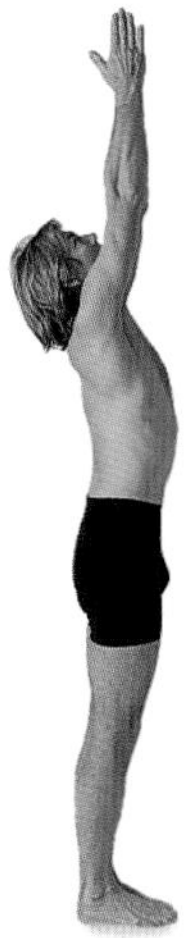

▲ 1 Ekam
Inhale

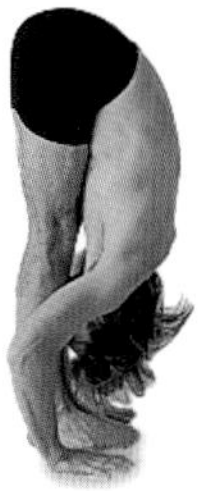

▲ 2 Dve
Exhale

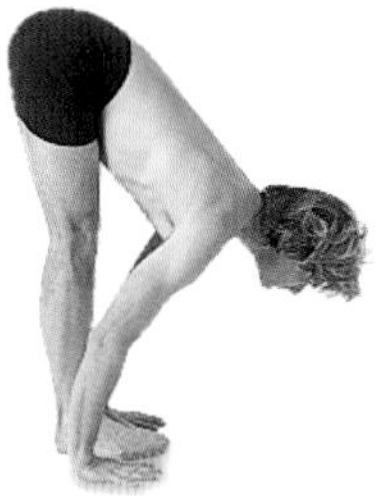

▲ 3 Trini
Inhale

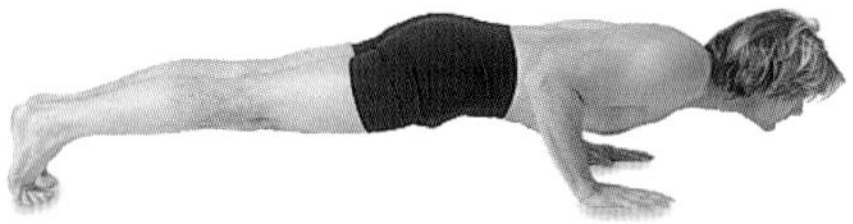

▲ 4 Chatvari
Exhale

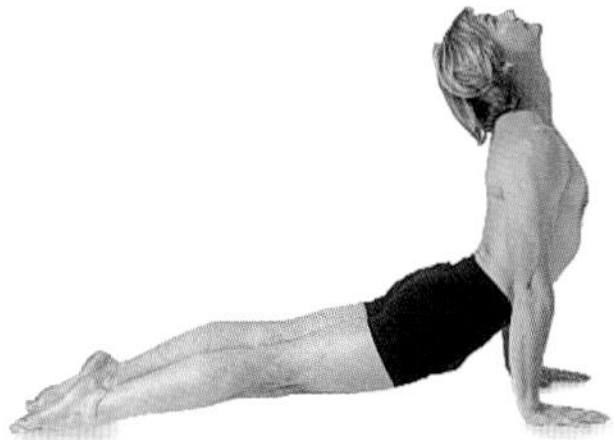

▲ 5 Panca
Inhale

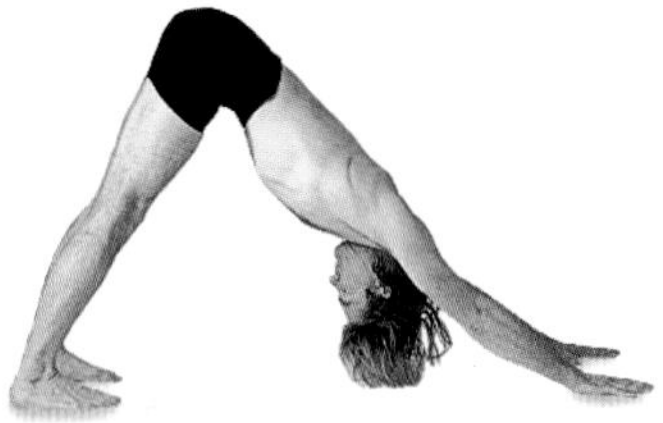

▲ 6 Shat
Exhale
(x 5 breaths)

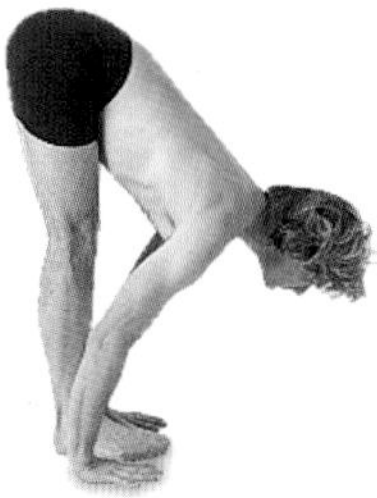

▲ 7 Sapta
Inhale

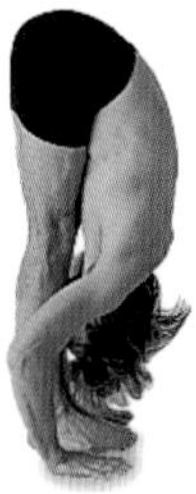

▲ 8 Ashtau
Exhale

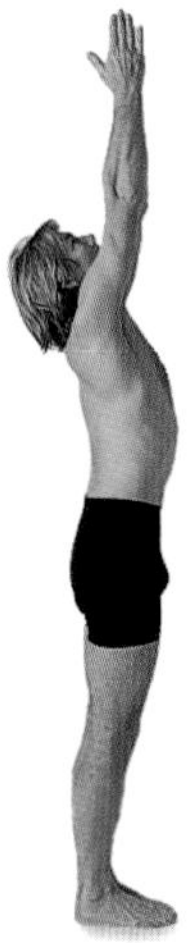

▲ 9 Nava
Inhale

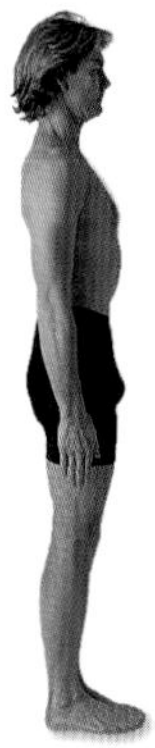

▲ Samasthitih
Exhale

Sun Salute B
Surya Namaskara B

Here, the attention to stretching the breath and bandhas helps to build internal heat, preparing the body for the move into Yoga Chikitsa.

Surya Namaskara B is repeated five times.

Samasthitih: Exhaling, stand in this neutral position, look to your nose.

1 Ekam: Inhaling, bend your knees, sit low, reach up, look to your thumbs.

2 Dve: Exhaling, forward bend, look to your nose.

3 Trini: Inhaling, lift your head, look to your third eye.

4 Chatvari: Exhaling, jump back, look to your nose.

5 Panca: Inhaling, roll to Upward-facing Dog, look to your third eye.

6 Shat: Exhaling, roll to Downward-facing Dog, look to your navel.

7 Sapta: Inhaling, turn your left heel in, step your right foot forward, bending your right knee 90°, hips square, reach up, look behind your thumbs.

8 Ashtau: Exhaling, hands on the mat either side of your right foot, step back (see step 4).

9 Nava: Inhaling, roll to Upward-facing Dog, look to your third eye.

10 Dasa: Exhaling, roll to Downward-facing Dog, look to your navel.

11 Ekadasa: Inhaling, turn your right heel in, step your left foot forward, bending the left knee 90°, hips square, reach up, look up behind your thumbs.

12 Dvadasa: Exhaling, hands on the mat either side of your left foot, step back (see step 4).

13 Trayodasa: Inhaling, roll to Upward-facing Dog, look to your third eye.

14 Chaturdasa: Exhaling, roll to Downward-facing Dog, look to your navel (5 breaths).

15 Pancadasa: Inhaling, jump up, look to your third eye.

16 Sodasa: Exhaling, forward bend, look to your nose.

17 Saptadasa: Inhaling, bend your knees, sit low, reach up, look to your thumbs.

Samasthitih: Exhaling, return to this neutral position, look to your nose.

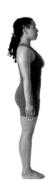
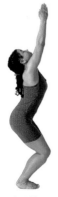
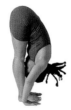

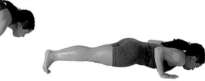

▲ **Samasthitih**
Exhale

▲ **1 Ekam**
Inhale

▲ **2 Dve**
Exhale

▲ **3 Trini**
Inhale

▲ **4 Chatvari**
Exhale

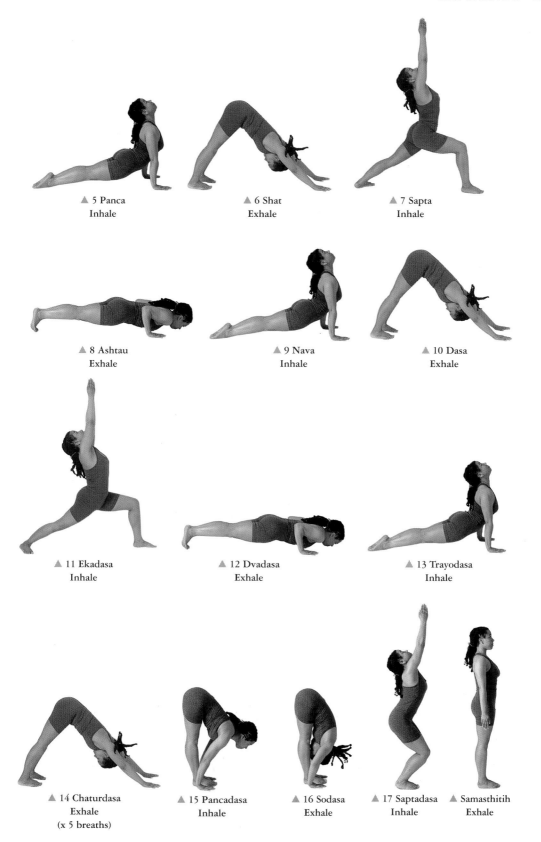

▲ 5 Panca
Inhale

▲ 6 Shat
Exhale

▲ 7 Sapta
Inhale

▲ 8 Ashtau
Exhale

▲ 9 Nava
Inhale

▲ 10 Dasa
Exhale

▲ 11 Ekadasa
Inhale

▲ 12 Dvadasa
Exhale

▲ 13 Trayodasa
Inhale

▲ 14 Chaturdasa
Exhale
(x 5 breaths)

▲ 15 Pancadasa
Inhale

▲ 16 Sodasa
Exhale

▲ 17 Saptadasa
Inhale

▲ Samasthitih
Exhale

Transitional Technique A

At first glance, these transitions, taken from Sun Salute A (*Surya Namaskara A – see pp. 24–5*), look like a simple routine to follow. However, beginners will very quickly discover many challenges here: how to fold forward without straining your lower back, for example, or how to transfer foundation and weight from your feet to your hands without falling forward, and how to synchronize your movement and breathing without holding or straining your breath. Transitional Technique A explores techniques to overcome these limitations. For the absolute beginner, additional variations are suggested where appropriate and you should also refer to the caution boxes. Established students will particularly benefit from the principles in steps 3 and 4.

caution
If you hold your breath in steps 3–5, tension will be created and you may jar your back on landing. Holding your breath also prevents energy flow and bandha control (see *pp. 20–3*). If you exhale, the transition is like floating.

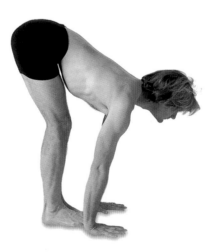

◀ 1 Exhaling
(Vinyasa 2) Bend your knees slightly and fold your torso forward, if possible placing your hands on the mat – don't overstretch your hamstrings. Check that your knees are facing forward and are parallel. If it helps, bend your knees a little more and place your hands forward of your feet. To work length into your hamstrings, distribute your body weight between your feet and hands. Then tip forward on to your hands and pull up on your quadriceps to straighten your legs as much as possible without straining your back.

◀ 2 Inhaling
(Vinyasa 3) With your hands a shoulder-width apart, middle fingers facing forward, press your hands into the mat. Lift your head and torso and look to the third eye dristi (see *p. 23*). Straighten your arms, but keep your hands on the mat as you tip your weight forward on to your hands. As you extend forward, try to lengthen the front line of your spine to create space between your ribcage and the top of your pelvis. Make this inhalation long and smooth, ready-ing yourself for the next exhalation.

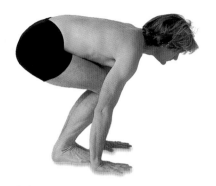

▲ 3 Exhaling

(Vinyasa 4) Initiate this transition with a long, flowing exhalation and bend right down into your knees, putting more weight on to your hands. As you tip forward, concentrate your gaze on a spot on the floor 30cm (12in) in front of your hands. Keep your arms as straight as possible. Check that your hands and feet are in the same positions as in step 2. This initial move should take about a third of your exhalation.

▼ 4 Still exhaling

(Vinyasa 4) With your body weight now in your hand foundation, jump your legs and bottom up. Push firmly into the mat, keeping your arms straight and your shoulders forward of your wrists. Your shoulder joints act as pivots so that as your bottom swings up, your head swings down. Keep your neck flexed and your gaze on the spot on the floor. To perfect this move, imagine there is an obstacle you are jumping your feet to avoid, or place a real obstacle about 30cm (12in) behind your feet. By placing an obstacle in your path, the only way past it is up.

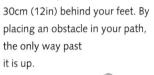

▲ 5 Still exhaling

(Vinyasa 4) From the "up" position, keep looking to your front. Jump your bottom and legs back while keeping your upper body forward. Land on the balls of your feet, feet a hip-distance apart. Jump too long or too short and the next transition will be difficult. In this "plank" position, your shoulders should be over your wrists. This and the previous two steps are executed on one continuous exhalation to activate uddiyana bandha (see pp. 22–3). Land with your bottom lifted just slightly above the ankle-to-shoulder line.

caution

If the jump back is too long in step 5, your shoulders will be behind your wrists and your upper body weight will not be supported, resulting in a collapse of the lumbar spine.

▶ 6 Inhaling

(Vinyasa 5) With a forward push, roll over your toes and point your feet back as much as possible. As you do this, bring your chest through your arms, forward of your hands. Keep your gaze down while lengthening through your spine from the sacrum to the base of the skull. Arch your back and then look forward and slightly up. Strongly work your legs, pulling up on your quadriceps to keep the front of your legs off the mat.

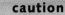

Transitional Technique B

In the beginning, it is common to lose the connective flow of breath, and the synchronicity of movement and breath. This sequence analyzes the two sections of Sun Salute B where the breath is commonly lost – the transitions into and out of the Warrior pose (vinyasas 6–7 and 7–8), and from the push-up position to the Upward-facing Dog (vinyasas 8–9). These transitions are demanding, and it is common for beginners to hold their breath, lose energy flow, and tense their muscles. When the energy flow stops, the elements of vinyasa are lost, and there is no cultivation of the inner body. Transitional Technique B looks at lengthening the exhalation so that it overlaps the next vinyasa, thus establishing the foundation for the coming inhalation. This overlap allows for a more complete inhalation. By stretching the breath, the correct vinyasa is maintained without taking extra breaths.

tip

In step 4, by looking to your foot, you can check your body alignment as you come into the Warrior. This also lengthens your neck while maintaining a quality inhalation. Don't look up until your hands are touching.

▶ **1 Exhaling**

(Vinyasa 6) From step 6, page 29, begin a long, controlled exhalation. Now lift through your bottom, roll back over your toes, and bring your upper torso and head through your arms to the Downward-facing Dog position. Although the correct dristi is your navel, look to your feet to prepare for your next foundation.

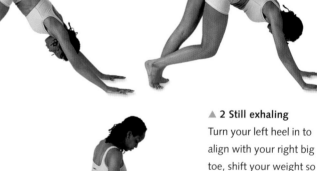

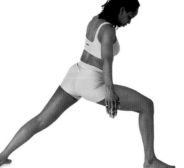

▲ **2 Still exhaling**

Turn your left heel in to align with your right big toe, shift your weight so that your foundation is transferred to your left foot, and prepare to step your right foot forward.

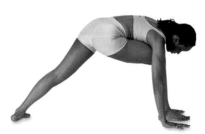

▲ **3 Still exhaling**

Stretching your exhalation just a little more, look ahead to the space between your hands. Transferring your weight fully on to your left foot, step your right foot as far forward as you can, aiming to place it beside your right thumb.

▲ **4 Inhaling**

(Vinyasa 7) As you release your hand foundation, sit into your pelvis and look to your right foot. Now begin to stand through your torso and start to raise your arms wide to the side. To finish the vinyasa, bring your hands together above your head and look to the sky.

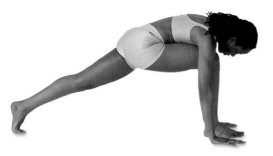

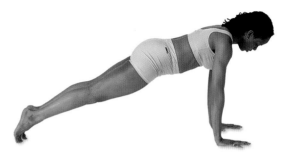

▲ **5 Exhaling**

(Vinyasa 8) Bring your hands back down to the mat and place them either side of your right foot, a shoulder-distance apart. Spread your fingers, the middle finger of each hand pointing directly forward. Turn on to the ball of your left foot and press firmly into your hands. Look to the space between your hands on the mat.

▲ **6 Still exhaling**

Step your right foot back so that it is a hip-distance from your left foot. Keep a strong lift through your pelvis and create a long, straight, inclined plane. Keep your arms straight and position your shoulders directly over your hands. Continue looking to the space between your hands.

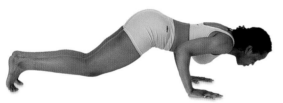

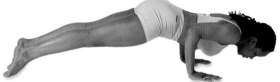

▲ **7 Still exhaling**

Keeping your elbows close in to your body, bend your elbows and lower yourself to about 5cm (2in) from the mat. Look to nasagrai dristi (see p. 23). Don't allow your body to go below the line of your upper arms. Complete novices can place their knees on the mat until they have developed the required strength in their upper body.

▲ **8 Still exhaling**

Stretching your exhalation just a little more, maintain the lift in your legs and bottom and roll over your toes to bring your shoulders forward, past the position of your hands.

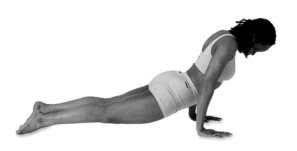

◀ **9 Inhaling**

(Vinyasa 9) Pressing firmly through your hands into the mat, begin to straighten your arms. Pull up on your kneecaps and thighs and point your toes. Relax your buttocks to prevent your lower back jamming up. Tuck your tailbone down, and lengthen your body through to your neck while continuing to look to nasagrai dristi. To finish, straighten your arms, lifting your sternum and rolling your shoulders back. Look to broomadhya dristi.

Beginner's Finishing
Padmasana

Padma means "lotus flower" – a beautiful description of this yoga position. The practice starts with you repeating the Sun Salutes (*Surya Namaskara*), weaving postures on the thread of the breath, like lacing daisies together to create a band. The lotus and resting positions are the final flowers that complete the circle.

At first, the Sun Salutes are demanding and you can quickly become short of breath. If you do, sit down on your mat in *Padmasana* and focus on ujjayi techniques to gain control (*see pp. 20–1*). Before placing your hands on your knees, hold your lower abdomen and "draw in" your abdominal wall to direct your breath up into your lungs and concentrate on the mula and uddiyana bandhas (*see pp 21–23*). When your breath is calm and your mind still, lie down and rest.

> **caution**
> Don't use your hands to pull your lower leg in, as this will stress your knee joint. Your hands must feel for the source of the movement coming from the hip joint. Synchronize this movement with an exhalation.

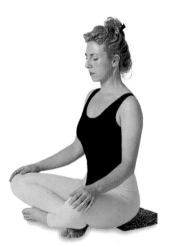

◀ Half-lotus variation

Sitting on a foam yoga block, inhale as you place your right leg into the lotus position. Take your thighbone well back to maximize the opening of your hips. Relax your calf muscle and bring your heel into your lower left abdomen, above the pubic bone. Your leg initiates this movement – use your hands only to position the foot. Now, exhale and fold your left leg under your right.

Sit tall, place your hands on your knees. Gaze to nasagrai dristi and focus on your ujjayi breathing and bandha techniques.

▲ Crossed-leg variation

Complete beginners can sit on the front edge of a foam block. Inhale, and then as you exhale fold your right leg, bringing your heel in toward your pubic bone. Inhale, and then as you exhale fold your left leg in, under your right. Allow your pelvis to rotate forward, off the front of the block. Lengthen your entire spine. Place your hands on your knees and gaze to nasagrai dristi. Breathe deeply and regulate your breath.

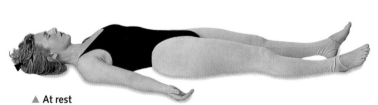

▲ At rest

Exhaling, release yourself from the lotus variation. Hold on to your bent legs and lower yourself down into the mat, one vertebra at a time, keeping your spine aligned. Release your legs and arms and allow your feet and hands to roll out to the sides. Close your eyes and let go of any tension with each exhalation.

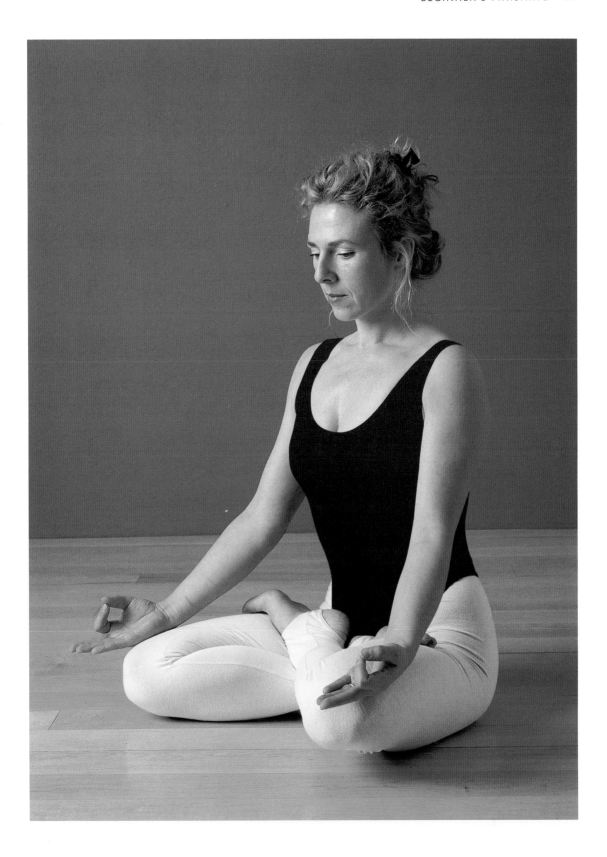

3

The Practice Session

The traditional method of learning the Ashtanga system of yoga was one to one – a single student working with his or her guru. Each asana, or posture, was given individually to the student when that student was deemed ready to receive it. More recently, however, two main methods of teaching have evolved. The first is the "Self-practice Method" in which the teacher introduces the practice, imparts information, monitors the individual's progress, and physically corrects the postures. The second is the "Traditional Counting Method", which is suited to students who have reached a level whereby they can practise the complete primary series, or Yoga Chikitsa (*see p. 15*) by themselves. The purpose of the counting method is to extend the breath so that the correct vinyasa can be achieved and to deepen the focus of individual practitioners. Through this, an understanding of the "complete" system develops. The understanding, experience, strength, and stamina gained from these two methods filters back into each individual's personal self-practice.

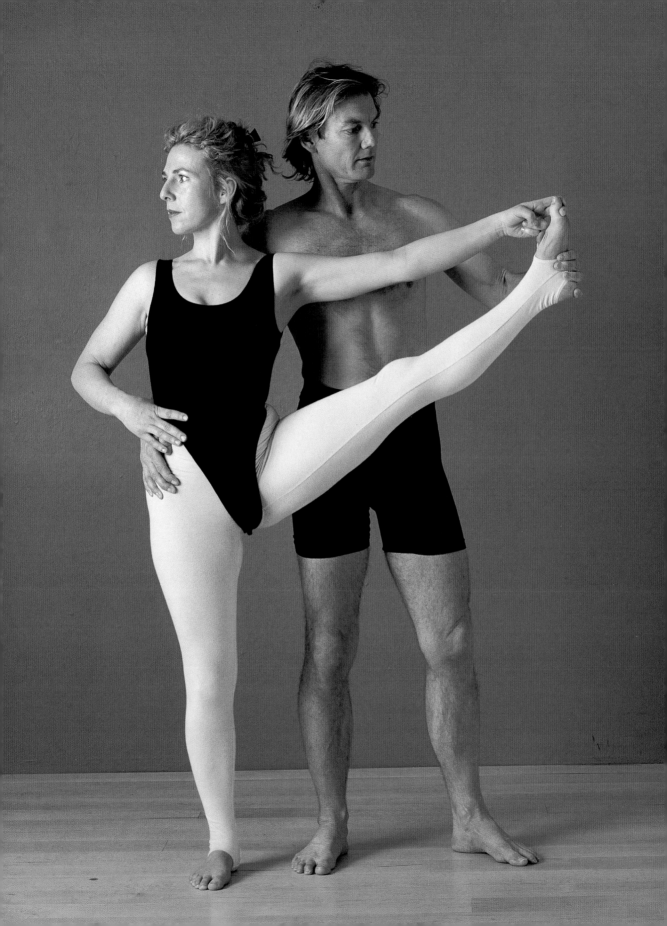

Sequence 1:

The Standing Sequence

Surya Namaskara A and *B*, which are commonly known as the Sun Salutes A and B (*see pp. 24–7*), have introduced the key vinyasa principles. From this core sequence of movements you should have gained some insight into the importance of the flowing repetition of the breath and the rhythm it creates. It is from this point that you establish the foundation for the entire practice that follows. The Sun Salutes have created the thread of the practice – it is now up to you to weave this thread into the sequence of standing postures that follow in order to continue the dynamic, meditative flow that is Ashtanga Yoga. Therefore, from the last exhalation of *Surya Namaskara B*, the first inhalation of the standing sequence begins. There is a counted number of vinyasas into and then out of each standing posture, always returning to *Samasthitih* (*see p. 38*).

The standing asanas explore our connection to the earth through our feet, how we work with the forces of gravity, to move, to balance, to find equilibrium. This is what is commonly referred to as "grounding". To create a dynamic standing posture, the techniques of vinyasa – the synchronicity of breath and movement (*see pp. 20–3*) – must all be present and in harmony, because it is through the control you exercise internally that the resultant external pose develops.

Through applying dristi gaze points, for example, your head will be in the correct relationship to your pelvis, and this, in turn, draws your focus inward to the breath and bandha (*see pp. 21–3*). The aim is to flow gracefully into the asana on the breath, exhaling into the posture to root yourself, as if into the earth itself. It is the mula bandha that establishes this root connection – through your legs and feet – like the anchors of a tree. Mula bandha provides the foundation for the correct position of your pelvis, and this is necessary since it is from this that the rest of the posture develops. Your inhalation supports uddiyana bandha, and it is the application of this bandha that provides the lightness and uplifting effect of your limbs.

From the strong foundation of your feet, which connect you down into the ground, you can draw in the earth's energy, bringing it upward and then directing it through your spinal column and outward to your limbs. It is interesting to discover that as the extension through your arms releases your shoulder joints and, simultaneously, the extension through your legs releases your hip joints, your spine becomes free, thus providing the space necessary for the correct alignment of your neck and pelvis.

In the standing poses, the alignment of your spine is also corrected through the application of the bandhas – uddiyana bandha equalizes the front and back of your spine, preventing any flaring of your ribcage and overarching of your back.

A secondary foundation, involving the hands, is also developed through the standing asanas. The supporting arm pushing into the ground helps to open your chest as well as provide an additional element of balance and support. It can be the element that completes an asana.

In the following standing sequences, the small-sized images are postures that have already been introduced and fully described, while the large ones depict a completed asana that you hold for a duration of five counted breaths. Bear in mind that Ashtanga Yoga is a continuously flowing sequence of movements, only briefly interrupted by a series of static asanas.

OPPOSITE *The group dynamics of Ashtanga Yoga are unique to its vinyasa system. The heat, the combined Victorious Breath, and the intense focus of the students produce a high-energy atmosphere.*

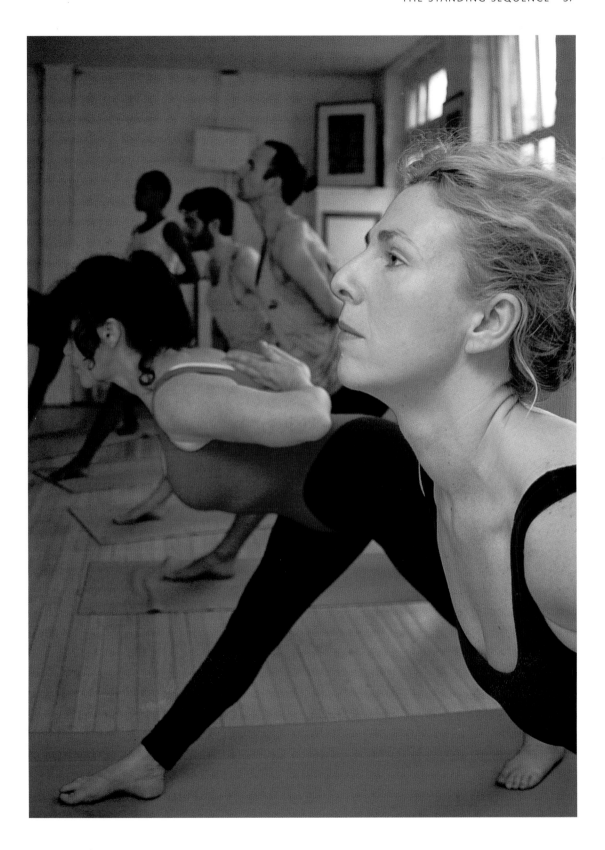

Sequence 1:
Standing Forward Bend A
Padangusthasana

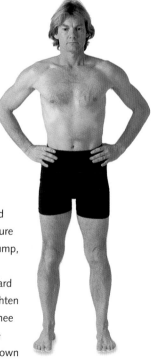

This is the first asana and it explores and applies the techniques that were previously outlined in the Sun Salutes, *Surya Namaskara* (*see pp. 24–7*). On entering and exiting *Padangusthasana*, place your hands on your lower abdomen to check for the correct application of uddiyana bandha (*see pp. 22–3*). For most beginners, the Standing Forward Bend highlights the concept "Form Follows Function", meaning that the form, or appearance, of a posture is governed by the range of functions, or movements, in the joints and muscles. To improve the application and depth of an asana, all your joints must move freely and be able to negotiate and perform the correct sequence of actions. The knee is the facilitator of this asana, supporting the limitations of the other joints (*see tip box*).

> **tip**
> In order to hold their big toes, beginners may have to bend their knees before they can access the function/mobility of their ankle and hip joints.

◀ 1 Exhaling
This pose, *Samasthitih*, begins and ends all the asanas. Standing tall, with big toe and ankle joints touching, pull up on your kneecaps and thighs. Level your pelvis by applying mula and uddiyana bandhas, root down into the floor, and lengthen upward through your spine. Relax your shoulders. With fingers together, align your hands with the centre of your thighs. Equilibrium comes from the balance between the right and left and front and back of your body.

▶ 2 Inhaling
In a fluid motion, bend your knees slightly and jump your feet a hip-distance apart, making sure your feet are parallel. Synchronous with the jump, place your hands on your waist to connect to uddiyana bandha and direct your breath upward to fill the space in your back and chest. Straighten your legs fully without over-extending your knee joints. Your hands should feel the result of the action of mula bandha, while your feet root down through the mat, creating a stable foundation.

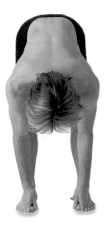

◀ 4 Inhaling

(Vinyasa 1) Press down through your big toe joints into the mat, holding your fingers. Extend your body forward, straightening your arms and lifting your spine and head. Look to the third eye dristi, or broomadhya (see p. 23). This lift is initiated from the breath and bandha. Straighten your legs while keeping your back and arms straight. This creates a powerful triangulation of circulating energy.

▲ 3 Exhaling

Maintain hand contact with your lower abdomen to ensure continued application of uddiyana bandha. Bend your knees slightly to access hip rotation, and fold your torso forward, rotating at the hip. Release your hands from uddiyana bandha and take hold of both big toes with your index and middle fingers.

◀ 5 Exhaling (x 5 breaths)

(Vinyasa 2) Release your knees a little to allow hip rotation and fold your torso over, bridging and maintaining the space in your lower abdomen created by the extension of uddiyana bandha. Pull up your kneecaps and thighs to straighten your legs to the extent your hamstrings will allow. Maintain a secure hold with your toes and fingers as your elbows move wide and back, creating a space between your shoulder blades. Gaze at the nasagrai dristi (see p. 23), hold this position and breathe deeply for five full breaths.

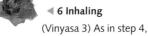

◀ 6 Inhaling

(Vinyasa 3) As in step 4, but on this inhalation create space between your pubic bone and sternum.

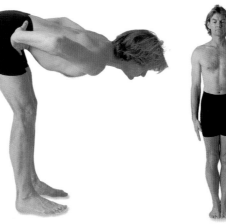

▶ 7 Exhaling

Maintaining the lift in the spine, make contact again with uddiyana bandha. Bend your knees slightly so that your leg muscles work to support the weight of your forward-leaning torso. Your torso is heavy in this position and the lumbar spine is at risk if your knees are locked out, so the bandha here is crucial to safeguard your lower back.

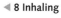

◀ 8 Inhaling

Come up, filling your chest and back with air, straighten your legs, and, exhaling fully, come back into Samasthitih. Lower your gaze point to nasagrai dristi.

Sequence 1:

Standing Forward Bend B
Padahastasana

In the Sanskrit name for this movement, *pada* translates as "foot" and *hasta* is the word for "hand". To perform this second forward bend you must stand fully on your hands – in essence, it is the same as *Padangusthasana (see pp. 38–9)*, except that here it is a little deeper. In this sequence, you need to pay attention to keeping a proper width between your shoulder blades in order to maintain the fullness of the ujjayi breath *(see pp. 18–21)*. Standing fully on your hands acts as a counterstretch to the wrist flexion required in vinyasa 3 of *Surya Namaskara* (Sun Salute). Allow yourself to tip your weight right into your hands and press with the back of your hands into the mat.

> **tip**
> A red face suggests blood is pooling in the neck and head due to a constriction of the shoulders and neck. To overcome this, and free the area, open your shoulders by drawing your elbows apart and back.

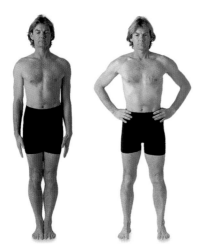

▲ **1–2 Exhaling–Inhaling**
As you exhale, stand with firm foundation in *Samasthitih (see p. 38)* – your gaze point is nasagrai dristi and your focus is mula bandha *(see pp. 21–2)*. You are now ready for the next inhalation. As you inhale, jump your feet a hip-distance apart and place your hands on uddiyana bandha.

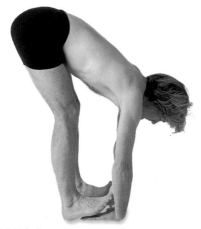

▲ **3 Exhaling**
Maintain hand contact with your lower abdomen in order to ensure the continued application of the protective uddiyana bandha. Bend your knees slightly and fold your torso forward from the hips. Release your hands from uddiyana bandha and place them fully under your feet. You will know that your hands are in the correct position when your toes touch your wrists. Your eyes should make a firm connection with the foundation where your feet and hands meet.

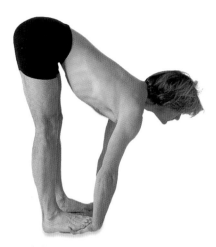

▲ 4 Inhaling
(Vinyasa 1) Pressing through the back of your hands, lift your spine until it is straight. Straighten your legs, look up to the third eye (broomadhya) dristi, and cultivate the length and extension of uddiyana bandha.

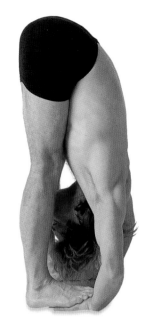

◀ 5 Exhaling (x 5 breaths)
(Vinyasa 2) Release your knees slightly to access hip rotation – you should feel as if you are folding over the space created by uddiyana bandha. Keeping your spine long and straight, bring your head down between your shins. Flex your knees and thighs to straighten your legs. Look to the nose (nasagrai) dristi Breathe deeply for five full breaths. Maintain your focus and control of the bandhas. Make sure you maximize and equalize the length of each inhalation and exhalation.

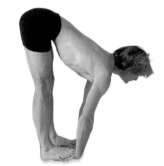

◀ 6 Inhaling
(Vinyasa 3) As in step 4, press through the back of your hands and look up to the third eye dristi. As you lengthen and lift your spine, feel the strength created by the triangulation of this position.

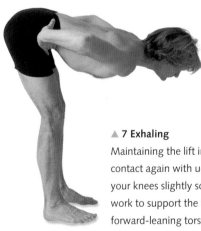

▲ 7 Exhaling
Maintaining the lift in the spine, make contact again with uddiyana bandha. Bend your knees slightly so that your leg muscles work to support the weight of your forward-leaning torso. Your torso is heavy in this position and the lumbar spine is at risk if your knees are locked out, so the bandha here is crucial to safeguard the lower back.

▶ 8 Inhaling
As you inhale, come up into a standing position and then, while you exhale, jump to *Samasthitih*.

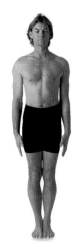

Sequence 1:

Triangle
Utthita Trikonasana

Utthita means "extended", *tri* translates as "three", and *kona* is "angle". The triangle posture challenges balance and alignment, and the use of the dristis (*see p. 23*) is essential in achieving a stable and firm foundation. This is the first asana that initiates the process of strengthening the legs and opening the hips. *Trikonasana* invigorates and strengthens the legs and helps to improve digestion, relieving constipation. Through the triangulation of your legs, torso, and the arm contacting your foot, your spine and neck are toned and stretched as you rotate your head to look up at the hand (hastagrai) dristi. Your legs have powerful work to do as your thighbones rotate away from one another, thus opening your hips. The hamstring of your leading leg is stretched as the underside of your torso lengthens away from the back of your hips. Your torso should remain as level as possible, and you need to activate the bandhas strongly (*see pp. 21–3*).

> **caution**
> Locking your knees creates excess weight loading on the knee joints, which may potentially lead to pain. To avoid this, bend your knees during transitions in order to work the muscles and not the ligaments.

◀ **2 Inhaling**
(Vinyasa 1) Jump to your right. Make sure that your feet are parallel (heels and arches aligned) and approximately 1m (3ft) apart. Raise your arms to shoulder height so that you feel the energy spread out to your fingertips – this enhances the opening of your shoulders, chest, and back. Uddiyana bandha supports your arms, like the wings of a great bird, but make sure that when you lift your arms your shoulders do not creep up toward your ears. Look straight ahead.

▲ **1 Exhaling**
As you exhale, stand with firm foundation in *Samasthitih* (*see p. 38*) – your gaze point is nasagrai dristi and your focus is mula bandha.

▶ **3 Exhaling**
(Vinyasa 2) Turn your right foot 90° and pivot your left foot slightly to the right. Turn your head to look at the fingers of your right hand . Release your right knee and bend to the right until your spine is parallel with the floor. Take hold of the right big toe with the first two fingers of your right hand.

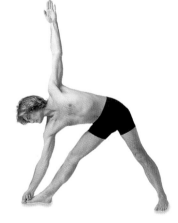

▼ 4 Inhaling (x 5 breaths)

Flex your knees and thighs to firm the foundation. Rotate your head and look up to the left hastagrai dristi. Breathe deeply for five full breaths, using the bandhas to align your spine over the foundation of your feet. Open your left hip, rotating your right buttock under, and stretch from the sacrum to the crown of your head. Continue to spread the energy out through your arms. Keep concentrating to avoid a collapse of your lower back. At the end of the last exhalation, slightly bend your right knee to protect it for the next transition.

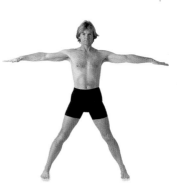

▲ 5 Inhaling

(Vinyasa 3) Initiating the lift with the bandhas, square your feet once again, as in step 2.

▶ 6 Exhaling

(Vinyasa 4) Turn your feet and head to the left and look to the fingers of your left hand. Then follow instructions as in step 3, changing right for left and left for right.

▶ 7 Inhaling (x 5 breaths)

Rotate your head, maintaining the line of the spine through your neck. Looking to the right hastagrai dristi helps to align the neck muscles. Firm your legs by contracting your quadriceps. Stretch the mat between your feet and roll your right hip open. By straightening the leading leg from a slightly bent position, hyperextension is avoided in the knee joint. Breathe deeply for five full breaths.

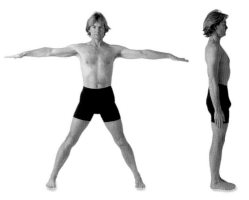

▲ 8–9 Inhaling–Exhaling

(Vinyasa 5) While inhaling, follow the directions in step 2 and, on the exhalation, jump back to the front of the mat and return to *Samasthitih*.

Sequence 1:

Revolving Triangle
Parivrtta Trikonasana

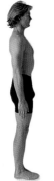

In the Sanskrit name for this asana, *parivrtta* means "revolving", while *tri* means "three", and *kona* translates as "angle". This rotating movement is the first spinal rotation in the primary series and you must take great care not to over-twist your body. This posture is stimulating and invigorating, benefiting your entire spine and nervous system. Your digestion is also improved by this asana due to the increase in digestive fire (*agni*), which burns up fats and helps to relieve constipation. This is the counterpose to the previous asana (*Utthita Trikonasana*).

> ### caution
> While performing this routine, don't go beyond your limits. If you feel any discomfort in your back, immediately stop twisting. As fitness and flexibility improve, you will be able to take the movement further.

◀ **2 Inhaling**
(Vinyasa 1) Jump to your right, legs apart and arms raised, and follow the instructions on page 42, step 2. Look straight ahead.

▲ **1 Exhaling**
Stand in *Samasthitih* (see p. 38). As you flow from asana to asana, *Samasthitih* becomes increasingly beneficial in centring your focus and equalizing your breath.

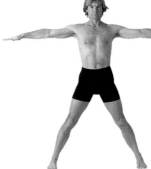

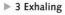

▶ **3 Exhaling**
(Vinyasa 2) Turn your feet to the right and face right. Rotate your whole body to the right, keeping your arms outstretched.
With your hips and shoulders directly in line with your leading leg, fold forward 90° so that your spine is parallel to the floor. Look to your right foot. The combination of outstretched arms and the temporary foot/floor dristi ensures good balance.

▲ **4 Still exhaling**
Now begin to "bank", like a bird – right wing up, left wing down. Your right arm provides lift while you place your left hand firmly on the mat beside your right foot. Your gaze is still on the floor. Limit rotation to the thoracic spine, keeping the lumbar spine extended and horizontal. Keep your pelvis square to the foundation.

◄ 5 Inhaling (x 5 breaths)

Pressing firmly on your left hand, turn your head to look up to your right hand. To complete the spinal twist, feel your left chest rotate through while your right chest opens to expand your ribcage. The lift in your right arm is important to prevent your left shoulder collapsing. Stretch the mat between your feet as you lengthen your spine and maintain a square foundation. Breathe deeply for five full breaths. At the end of the last exhalation, bend your right knee slightly to protect it for the transition to follow.

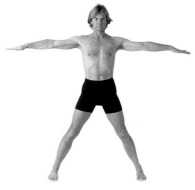

▲ 6 Inhaling

(Vinyasa 3) Come up, arms still outstretched, as in step 2.

◄ 8 Still exhaling

This is the reverse of step 4, with an intermediate dristi of looking to the front foot. The smooth-flowing exhalation enhances bandha control, supporting the lumbar region of the spine and the rooting of the feet into the mat. Keep your knees fluid.

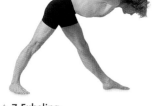

▲ 7 Exhaling

(Vinyasa 4) Turn your feet to the left and rotate around and down to the flying position – see step 3.

► 9 Inhaling (x 5 breaths)

Press firmly on your right hand and turn your head to look up to your raised left hand, then follow instructions in step 5. Breathe deeply for five full breaths. Although the twist is in the thoracic spine, the spine from the sacrum to the crown of the head is stretched.

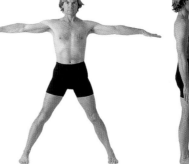

▲ 10–11 Inhaling–Exhaling

(Vinyasa 5) While inhaling, follow the directions in step 2 and, on the exhalation, jump back to the front of the mat and return to *Samasthitih*.

Sequence 1:

Lateral Angle
Utthita Parsvakonasana

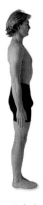

Utthita can be translated as "extended", *parsva* as "to the side", and *kona* as "angle". This dynamic sideways stretch is a powerful position, which is a variation of *Virabhadrasana*, or Warrior Sequence (*see pp. 66–7*), and encourages a complete stretch of your groin and spine. While your legs work in a semi-lunge position to support your entire body, your spine is kept in a straight line. This line of energy, running from the outer edge of your back foot right to the tips of your fingers, can be likened to the spear of the warrior – the energy moves from your foot up to your extended hand. The opposing force of the knee into the supporting arm helps to maintain the correct leg alignment and foundation, facilitating the opening of the groin.

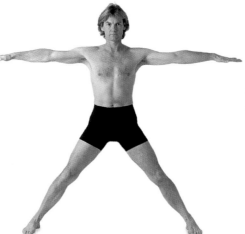

◀ 2 Inhaling
(Vinyasa 1) Jump to the right – as in step 2, page 42. The only difference here is that your feet need to be slightly wider apart – about 1.2m (4ft).

▲ 1 Exhaling
As you exhale, stand with firm foundation in *Samasthitih* (*see p. 38*) – your gaze point is nasagrai dristi and your focus is mula bandha.

▶ 3 Exhaling
(Vinyasa 2) Turn your right foot out 90°. Keeping your spine vertical, turn your head to focus on your right hand as you bend your right knee 90°. Your knee should be directly over the middle of your foot. Extend your spine to the right and place the palm of your right hand flat on the mat on the outside of your right foot. Your right knee presses firmly into your right armpit as your left arm extends upward to keep the chest open.

◄ 4 Inhaling (x 5 breaths)

Rotate your extended arm to bring it over your head, creating a long, straight line from the outer edge of your left foot to the tip of your left fingers. Rotate your head toward your armpit and look along your arm to the left hastagrai dristi. Use the opposing force between your right knee and right arm to roll open your left chest, abdomen, hip, and thigh. Keep both sides of your ribcage as equal as possible and guard against arching your back by tucking your tailbone down as you draw your abdomen in strongly (uddiyana bandha). Breathe deeply for five full breaths.

▶ 5 Inhaling

(Vinyasa 3) Return to the outstretched arms position of step 2.

◄ 6 Exhaling

(Vinyasa 4) To work the other side of your body, follow the instructions of step 3, reversing the left and right directions. Take care to maintain the correct distance between your feet and keep your spine vertical while you move down into the posture.

▶ 7 Inhaling (x 5 breaths)

Rotating your right shoulder joint, bring your arm over, as in step 4. This action is similar to an overarm tennis serve – imagine the ball is out of reach and maintain the extension you would need to try and hit it. Guard against flaring your ribs – this will close the area between your shoulder and neck. This area should remain open and soft. Rotate through your spine and turn your head toward your armpit to look along your arm to your right hastagrai dristi. Breathe deeply for five full breaths.

▲ 8–9 Inhaling–Exhaling

(Vinyasa 5) Inhale as you slowly come up, turning your feet parallel once more. As you exhale, jump to the front of the mat and return to *Samasthitih*.

Sequence 1:

Revolving Lateral Angle
Parivrtta Parsvakonasana

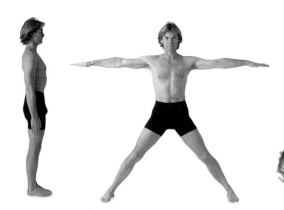

Parivrtta means "revolving", *parsva* "to the side", and *kona* translates as "angle". This revolving asana is the second spinal rotation in the primary series, and you require greater control of your breath if you are to perform it correctly. The first five standing asanas continue to develop the principles introduced in the Sun Salutes (*see pp. 24–7*), but here, in *Parivrtta Parsvakonasana*, the powerful twist involved in the routine stretches the development of breath/bandha integration (*see pp. 20–3*). The challenge in this asana is to twist fully down into the foundation as you exhale, without taking extra breaths, and then to maintain a constant, even flow of unrestricted breath. The development of mula and uddiyana bandhas will direct the breath into your lungs and thereby encourage expansion of your ribcage.

▼ 3 Exhaling
(Vinyasa 2) Turn your right foot out 90° and your left foot in slightly. Turn your head to focus on your right hand as you bend your knee 90°. Place your right hand on the side of your right thigh and, leading with your elbow, rotate around with your left arm to a point past the centre line of your right thigh. Using the leverage of your right hand against the foundation of your right thigh, completely twist and lengthen your thoracic spine while maintaining length in your lumbar spine.

▲ 1–2 Exhaling–Inhaling
As you exhale, stand with firm foundation in *Samasthitih* (*see p. 38*). Then (Vinyasa 1), inhaling, jump to the right – as in step 2, page 46.

◀ 4 Still exhaling
(Vinyasa 2) Continuing the pressure against your thigh, fold and rotate right down until the armpit of your left arm rests on your right thigh. Straighten and twist your left arm down and place your left hand flat into the mat. Release your right arm from supporting your thigh and straighten, ready to rotate over. Press down into your left foot and sit into your pelvis.

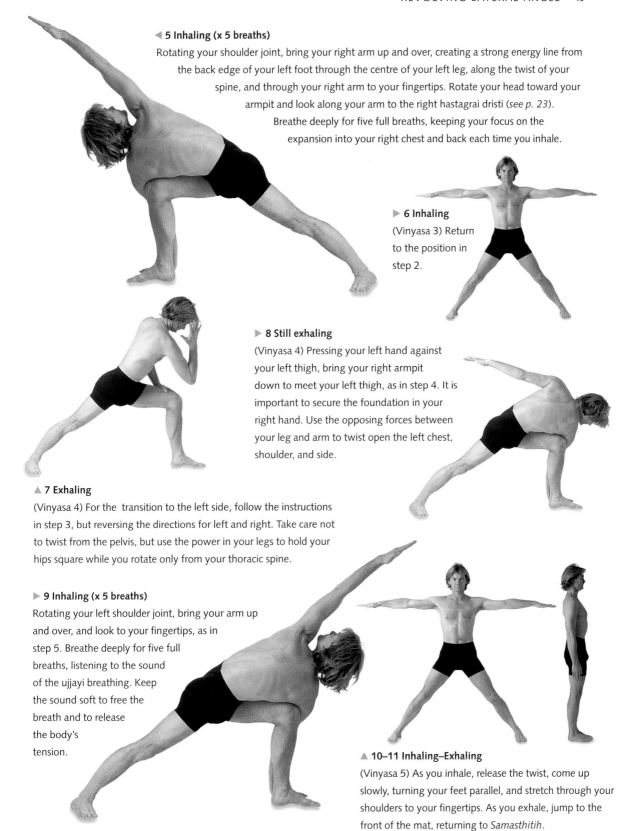

◀ **5 Inhaling (x 5 breaths)**
Rotating your shoulder joint, bring your right arm up and over, creating a strong energy line from the back edge of your left foot through the centre of your left leg, along the twist of your spine, and through your right arm to your fingertips. Rotate your head toward your armpit and look along your arm to the right hastagrai dristi (*see p. 23*). Breathe deeply for five full breaths, keeping your focus on the expansion into your right chest and back each time you inhale.

▶ **6 Inhaling**
(Vinyasa 3) Return to the position in step 2.

▶ **8 Still exhaling**
(Vinyasa 4) Pressing your left hand against your left thigh, bring your right armpit down to meet your left thigh, as in step 4. It is important to secure the foundation in your right hand. Use the opposing forces between your leg and arm to twist open the left chest, shoulder, and side.

▲ **7 Exhaling**
(Vinyasa 4) For the transition to the left side, follow the instructions in step 3, but reversing the directions for left and right. Take care not to twist from the pelvis, but use the power in your legs to hold your hips square while you rotate only from your thoracic spine.

▶ **9 Inhaling (x 5 breaths)**
Rotating your left shoulder joint, bring your arm up and over, and look to your fingertips, as in step 5. Breathe deeply for five full breaths, listening to the sound of the ujjayi breathing. Keep the sound soft to free the breath and to release the body's tension.

▲ **10–11 Inhaling–Exhaling**
(Vinyasa 5) As you inhale, release the twist, come up slowly, turning your feet parallel, and stretch through your shoulders to your fingertips. As you exhale, jump to the front of the mat, returning to *Samasthitih*.

Sequence 1:

Sideways Stretch A
Prasarita Padottanasana A

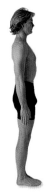

The word *prasarita* means "spread out", *pada* translates as "foot", and *uttana* is "intense stretch". This wide leg stretch is similar to the Standing Forward Bend we have already seen (*see pp. 38–9*), but here beginners may need some assistance to help them place their head on the mat without losing balance and falling over. This asana is, therefore, a good gauge for assessing just how flexible you have become. If, for example, you have limited rotation in your hip joints and you do require assistance, then this is an indicator that you should stop – do not progress through the practice session any further until you can complete this asana without any help at all. *Prasarita Padottanasana* has four variations – A, B, C, and D (*see also pp. 52–7*) – each with five vinyasas (breath-synchronized movements).

tip
Within each of these sequences there is an uncounted position designed specifically to cultivate bandha control (*see pp. 21–3*).

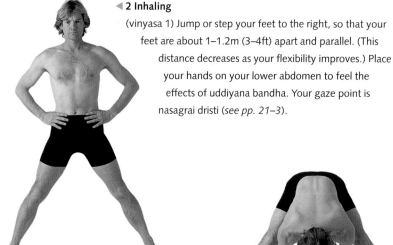

◀ 2 Inhaling
(vinyasa 1) Jump or step your feet to the right, so that your feet are about 1–1.2m (3–4ft) apart and parallel. (This distance decreases as your flexibility improves.) Place your hands on your lower abdomen to feel the effects of uddiyana bandha. Your gaze point is nasagrai dristi (*see pp. 21–3*).

▲ 1 Exhaling
As you exhale, stand with firm foundation in *Samasthitih* (*see p. 38*).

▶ 3 Exhaling
(Vinyasa 2) Bend your knees slightly and fold your torso forward at the hip joints so that you can place your hands a shoulder-distance apart on the mat. Look at the placement of your hands – if you are a beginner, your hands can be forward of your toes, although eventually your fingers and toes should line up.

◀ **4 Inhaling**

Pressing firmly through your hands, straighten your arms, and look to your third eye dristi or to the horizon. Using the strength in your breath and bandhas to lengthen the front line of your spine, straighten and work your quadriceps strongly. Do not collapse or overarch your lower back.

▶ **5 Exhaling (x 5 breaths)**

(Vinyasa 3) Bend your knees slightly to release your hip and ankle joints. The flexion in your ankles allows you to fold forward, tipping the weight of your torso into your hands. Bending at your elbows, place the crown of your head down into the mat. At the beginning, your head will be forward of your hands, but eventually you will be able to place your head comfortably between your hands. Gaze to the nasagrai dristi and breathe deeply for five full breaths.

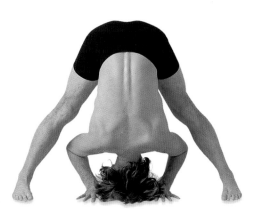

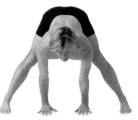

▲ **6 Inhaling**

(Vinyasa 4) Return to the position described in step 4.

◀ **7 Exhaling**

Maintaining the lift in your spine, release your hands from the mat and make contact again with uddiyana bandha. Bend your knees slightly so that your leg muscles work to support the weight of your forward-leaning torso. The combination of your bent knees and the application of uddiyana bandha will protect your lower back in the next transition.

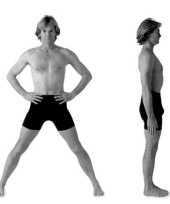

◀ **8–9 Inhaling–Exhaling**

While inhaling, maintain contact with uddiyana bandha as you follow the directions in step 2. On the exhalation, jump back to the front of the mat and return to *Samasthitih*.

Sequence 1:

Sideways Stretch B
Prasarita Padottanasana B

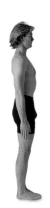

In this, *Prasarita Padottanasana B*, the second of the sideways stretch routines, it is possible to feel if you are achieving the correct application of uddiyana bandha (*see pp. 22–3*) because your hands remain resting on your lower abdomen throughout the whole sequence. If you try to muscle your way through this asana, your abdominal wall will harden, leading to a shortening of the distance between your sternum and pubic bone. This shortening acts to restrict the depth and power of your inhalation and then tension from your abdomen will spread to the rest of your body. As the cascade of problems continues, your legs will go hard and then this stiffness is referred into the region of your lower back. To avoid all of this, you need to feel for the subtlety of uddiyana bandha. This will give you the security you need to relax your abdominal wall, and this, in turn, leads to a releasing and lengthening of your lower back.

tip
By turning your toes slightly inward, as shown in step 5 opposite, you can establish a stronger foundation, and this in turn helps you to roll your thighs out.

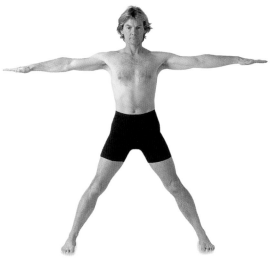

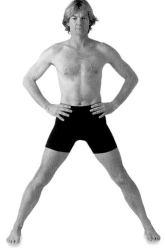

▲ **1 Exhaling**
As you exhale, stand with firm foundation in *Samasthitih* (*see p. 38*).

▲ **2 Inhaling**
(Vinyasa 1) Jump your feet to the right, so that they are 1–1.2m (3–4ft) apart and parallel – this variation is a little more difficult than the A version (*see pp. 50–1*), so your feet placement can be wider if necessary. As you jump, extend your arms wide, parallel to the floor. Controlling your bandhas, direct your inhalation upward and feel the internal energy flow out through your fingertips. Look straight ahead to the horizon.

▲ **3 Exhaling**
(Vinyasa 2) Bring your hands down to your lower abdomen to feel your uddiyana bandha. This position is the same as step 2, page 50, except that here you are feeling the effects of uddiyana bandha on an exhalation instead of an inhalation. Bring your gaze in, to the tip of your nose.

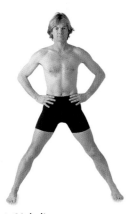

◄ 4 Inhaling

Keeping in contact with your uddiyana bandha, open your chest and heart. Don't overstretch, thereby pushing your sacrum and tailbone out. Concentrate instead on tucking your tailbone down, lengthening your lumbar spine as you firm your quadriceps. As you maintain the length in the back of your neck, look up to your third eye dristi (see p. 23), or to the sky.

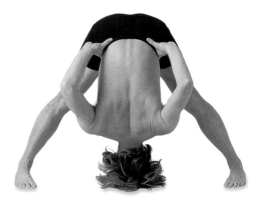

▲ 5 Exhaling (x 5 breaths)

(Vinyasa 3) Bend your knees slightly and fold forward at your hip joints. Place your head on the mat between your feet. Look again to nasagrai dristi and breathe deeply for five full breaths, continuing to feel the relationship between your breath and uddiyana bandha. If your head does not reach the floor, bend your knees a little more. Then, taking a little weight through your head, straighten your legs. As you do this, try and roll your quadriceps out, up to the sky.

▲ 6 Inhaling

(Vinyasa 4) Bend your knees slightly and return to the position in step 3. But this time, look at your nose dristi or straight ahead. Make sure your feet are parallel and pull up on your kneecaps and thighs.

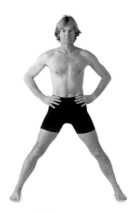

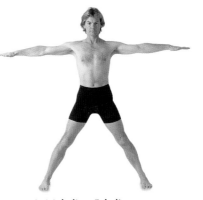

▲ 7 Exhaling

Remain in this position – hands on bandha – for the full exhalation. Keep the foundation in your legs strong and check your uddiyana bandha.

▲ 8–9 Inhaling–Exhaling

(Vinyasa 5) Open your arms wide to shoulder height as you inhale and feel the energy rise up through your body and out your fingertips. As you exhale, jump to the front of the mat, returning to *Samasthitih*.

Sequence 1:

Sideways Stretch C
Prasarita Padottanasana C

In *Prasarita Padottanasana C*, the third of the sideways stretches, you need to link your hands behind your back. It is this "tying up" of your hands that makes this the most difficult of the four variations. The first two have prepared you by bringing your attention to uddiyana bandha (*see pp. 21–3*). Here, it is crucially important to follow the principle of "Form Follows Function" (*see p. 38*) to avoid falling. By using the correct bandha control, you will be able to rotate your torso down confidently, placing your head on the mat and "hanging" from your hips. The correct application of mula bandha will root your legs down into the mat for a secure foundation, while uddiyana bandha will release your hip joints and allow you to free your shoulder joints to rotate your arms over and down to the mat.

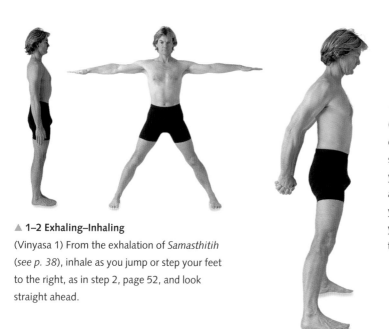

▲ 1–2 Exhaling–Inhaling
(Vinyasa 1) From the exhalation of *Samasthitih* (*see p. 38*), inhale as you jump or step your feet to the right, as in step 2, page 52, and look straight ahead.

◀ 3 Exhaling
(Vinyasa 2) Maintaining the extension in your arms, rotate your shoulder joints forward and bring your hands down behind your back and clasp them together. Straighten your arms to lift them away from your bottom and bring your gaze in, to the tip of your nose.

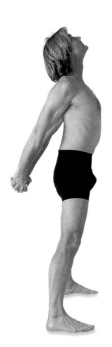

◀ 4 Inhaling

Now, roll your shoulders backward, opening your chest through your sternum and heart. Lift your arms as high as possible, tuck your tailbone down, and arch up to lengthen your whole spine. Don't let your head drop back – this will "jam" the back of your neck and restrict your inhalation. Straighten your legs and change your gaze to your third eye dristi, or to the sky.

▶ 5 Exhaling (x 5 breaths)

(Vinyasa 3) Bend your knees slightly, fold forward at your hips, and place your head on the mat between your feet. Tuck your chin in toward your sternum and bring your arms down to the floor behind you. Straighten your legs. Now look to nasagrai dristi and breathe deeply for five full breaths. Keep your focus on the rhythm of your breath – the free-flowing ujjayi breath (*see pp. 18–21*) and the connection to your bandhas enable you to maintain balance without falling over while you release your shoulder joints and ease your arms to the floor.

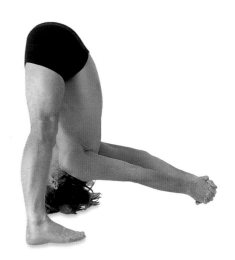

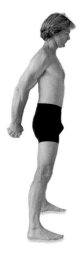

▲ 6 Inhaling–Exhaling

(Vinyasa 4) Inhaling, keep your hands clasped together, slightly bend your knees, and return to the position in step 3. Remain in this clasped-hand position as you exhale fully. Continue working your legs and lower your gaze to straight ahead.

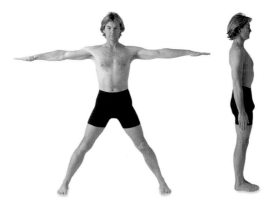

▲ 7–8 Inhaling–Exhaling

(Vinyasa 5) Open your arms wide to shoulder height as you inhale and feel the energy rise up through your body and out your fingertips. As you exhale, jump to the front of the mat, returning to *Samasthitih*.

Sequence 1:

Sideways Stretch D
Prasarita Padottanasana D

Through the repetition of the three preceding variations of *Prasarita Padottanasana* (*see pp. 50–5*), your hip joints and legs have undergone a very powerful stretching experience. In this routine, the final variation of sideways stretching, you can move your legs a little closer together in order to enjoy a still-deeper stretch. The final distance between your feet will be governed by the relationship of the length of your spine with the flexibility of your hip joints. The more open your hips joints become, the closer together your feet can be. The internal strength from your bandha control (*see pp. 21–3*) will eventually allow you to fold completely in half without having to rely on your head to support any of your weight.

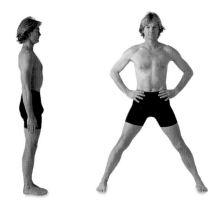

▲ **1–2 Exhaling–Inhaling**

(Vinyasa 1) From the exhalation of *Samasthitih* (*see p. 38*), inhale as you jump or step your feet to the right, as in step 2, page 52, and look straight ahead.

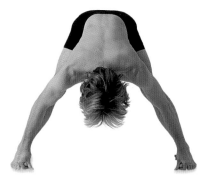

▲ **3 Exhaling**

(Vinyasa 2) Bend your knees slightly, fold your torso forward at the hip joints, and grasp your big toes with the first two fingers of each hand. The correct hold is to slip your first two fingers between your big toe and second toe and then press your thumb into the mat.

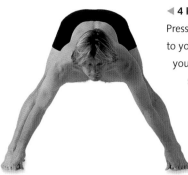

◀ 4 Inhaling

Pressing through your thumbs, straighten your arms and look to your third eye dristi, or to the horizon. Use the strength in your breath and bandhas to lengthen the front line of your spine. Straighten and work your quadriceps strongly. Do not collapse or overarch your lower back, and do not look up too high – this will cause you to "jam" the back of your neck.

▶ 5 Exhaling (x 5 breaths)

(Vinyasa 3) Once again, bend your knees slightly to release your hip and ankle joints. Bending your elbows, fold forward, tipping your weight over on to your strong foot foundation. Place the crown of your head down so that it just lightly touches the mat. Try and align your head with your feet. Strongly activate your quadriceps, rolling your thighs upward so that you feel as if you are stretching the mat between your feet. Gaze to the nasagrai dristi and breathe deeply for five full breaths.

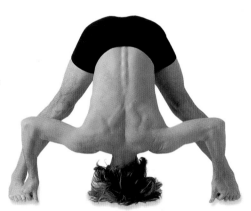

◀ 6 Inhaling

(Vinyasa 4) Pressing through your thumbs, straighten your arms and look to your third eye dristi, or to the horizon – as in step 4.

▶ 7 Exhaling

Maintaining the lift in your spine, release your hands from the mat, making contact again with uddiyana bandha. Bend your knees slightly so that your leg muscles work to support the weight of your forward-leaning torso. The combination of bent knees and uddiyana bandha will protect your lower back in the next transition.

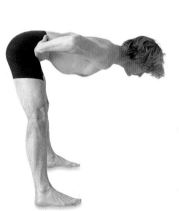

▲ 8 & 9 Inhaling–Exhaling

While inhaling, maintain contact with uddiyana bandha as you follow the directions in step 2. On the exhalation, jump back to the front of the mat and return to *Samasthitih*.

Sequence 1:
Side Forward Bend
Parsvottanasana

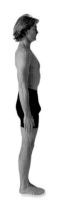

Parsva translates as "to the side", while *uttana* means "intense stretch". This standing forward bend is the necessary precursor to the standing leg raises that follow (*see pp. 60–1*), preparing you as it does for the foundation to be transferred to only one leg. Here, your hips are held square and level by the position of your back leg, while your torso is stretched over your front leg. Your arms are taken up behind you, pressed firmly together in the reverse prayer position, and the pressure from your hands promotes a straightening of the spine. This reverse prayer position also acts to open your shoulder joints, and this, together with the pressure into your spine, opens up your chest to allow you to stretch deeply over your forward-positioned leg. The hamstring of your forward leg is then intensely stretched.

▲ 1 Exhaling
Stand with firm foundation in *Samasthitih* (*see p. 38*).

◀ 2 Inhaling
(Vinyasa 1) Jump your feet to the right so that they are 60–90cm (23–36in) apart and parallel. As you jump, bring your arms around behind you and roll your shoulders forward. Slide the backs of your hands up your back until the outer edges of your little fingers touch. Then press your palms firmly together with the little fingers aligned with your thoracic spine. Look straight ahead.

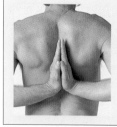

Bare skin is best for this position, with a little sweat to lubricate your hands as you slide them up your spine. Pressing your palms firmly together and into your spine releases tension in your shoulders and opens up the heart region.

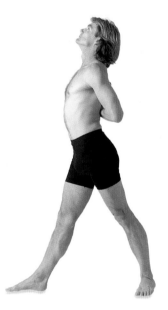

▲ 3 Still inhaling
Turn your right foot out to 90°. Initiate this from your right hip and roll your whole leg out to align the thigh, knee, shin, and foot. Turn your hips to face directly in line with your right leg. Press your hands into your thoracic spine and arch upward, opening the heart. Look up to your third eye dristi.

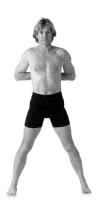

◀ 4 Exhaling (x 5 breaths)

(Vinyasa 2) Bend your right knee slightly and fold over your right leg. With the sensation of stretching the mat between your feet, pull up your kneecaps and thighs. To promote a lengthening out of the front body, direct the pressure of your hands toward your head. Now align your torso along your right leg. Gaze to the padhayoragrai dristi (see p. 23) and breathe deeply for five full breaths.

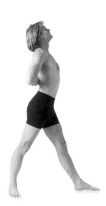

▲ 5–6 Inhaling

(Vinyasa 3) Return to the position shown in step 2, and then turn to your left following the instructions in step 3, reversing the directions for right and left. Take care when you turn to keep your heels aligned, and when you arch your back keep your tailbone well tucked in.

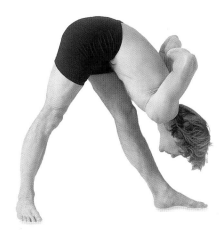

▲ 7 Exhaling (x 5 breaths)

(Vinyasa 4) Bend your left knee slightly to access the full rotation of the pelvis and fold over your left leg, as in step 4. Gaze to the padhayoragrai dristi and breathe deeply for five full breaths. Focus on the sole of your front foot, working strongly from your big toe joint to your hip joint to maintain square and level hips. Extend forward from your heart region and lengthen your ribs away from your pelvis to maintain strong bandha control.

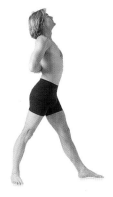
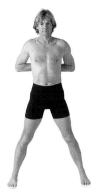
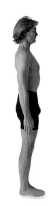

▲ 8–9–10 Inhaling–Exhaling

(Vinyasa 5) Inhale as you slowly come up to the positions described in steps 6 and then 5, turning your feet so that they are parallel once more. As you exhale, jump to the front of the mat and return to *Samasthitih*.

Sequence 1:
Standing Leg Raises
Utthita Hasta Padangusthasana

Utthita means "extended", *hasta* translates as "hand", and *padangustha* is "big toe". This dynamic pose is the first time that you will be standing wholly on one limb. The bandhas (*see pp. 21–3*) are necessary to keep the pose centralized and your free hand rests on uddiyana bandha to check and maintain it. Once again, your hips must be level while only the raised leg moves from the front to the side and then back to the front. Your head moves with the gaze point, or dristi, to counterbalance the leg when it is raised to the side. Your torso, however, remains centred throughout and the foot that you stand on acts as the foundation for the whole body. Elements of work from all the previous standing asanas support this sequence.

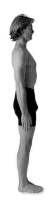

▲ 1 Exhaling
Stand with firm foundation in *Samasthitih* (*see p. 38*).

◀ 2 Inhaling
Extend your gaze point from the tip of your nose to a spot on the floor about 3.5m (12ft) away. Place your hands on your lower abdomen to connect with uddiyana bandha and slightly bend your left knee. Now transfer your body weight on to your left leg by lifting your right heel just off the floor.

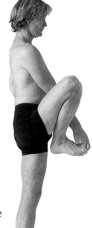

▶ 3 Exhaling
Bend your right leg up and catch the big toe with the first two fingers of your right hand (the toe also holds your fingers). Pull up on the kneecap and thigh of your left leg and stand tall up through your spine.

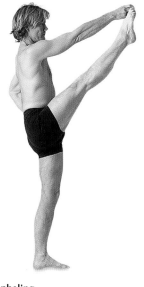

▲ 4 Inhaling
(Vinyasa 1) Feeling a strong foundation in your left standing leg, and keeping your hips square and level, straighten your right leg, lifting your toes to eye level. Pointing your big toe helps to direct your leg upward. Resisting this movement with your right arm helps to keep your shoulders square. If your balance is secure, then change your gaze to your toes.

◀ **6 Inhaling**
(Vinyasa 3) Lift your torso back, away from your raised leg, and stand tall – as in step 4.

◀ **5 Exhaling (x 5 breaths)**
(Vinyasa 2) Using the opposing forces existing between your standing and raised legs, bend your right elbow and draw your torso into the raised leg, touching your chin to your shin. Keep your left hand on your waist to help focus on uddiyana bandha and extend forward along your raised leg. Look to padhayoragrai (toes) dristi (*see p. 23*). Breathe deeply for five full breaths.

▶ **7 Exhaling (x 5 breaths)**
(Vinyasa 4) Maintaining the foundation through your standing leg and spine, move your raised leg to the right. Again, mula and uddiyana bandhas secure your pelvis and leg foundation. Don't lift your right hip – this causes your lower back to jam. Continue to point your big toe and resist with your fingers. Now look to your left side, finding a spot on the wall or floor as far left as possible. This is parsva dristi. Breathe deeply for five full breaths.

◀ **8 Inhaling–Exhaling**
(Vinyasa 5) Swing your raised leg back to the front and follow the instructions for step 4. Then, exhaling (vinyasa 6), fold forward again, chin to shin, as in step 5.

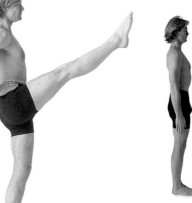

▶ **9 Inhaling (x 5 breaths)**
(Vinyasa 7) Stand tall once again, continuing to extend out through your raised leg. Release your fingers from your big toe and bring your right hand down to your lower abdomen. Hold your uddiyana bandha tight with both hands and send your internal energy out to your pointed toes. Maintaining your hands-free leg lift, breathe deeply for five full breaths while gazing to padhayoragrai dristi.

▲ **10 Exhaling**
Exhale as you slowly lower your leg, returning to *Samasthitih*. Then repeat all these steps for your other leg, reversing the instructions for left and right vinyasas.

Sequence 1:

Half-lotus Bound, Standing Forward Bend
Ardha Baddha Padmottanhasana

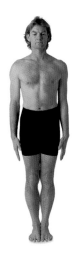

Ardha is the Sanskrit word for "half", *baddha* translates as "bound", *padma* means "lotus", and *uttana* is an "intense stretch". This particular forward bend is the first of the standing bound asanas. This is significant as the internal cleansing process occurring in the standing asanas is intensified with the binding of the lotus as demonstrated in this posture. The blood supply to the bound leg and arm is considerably reduced, and during the forward bend the heel of the folded leg presses into the spleen and liver, respectively. When you release from the posture, fresh oxygenated blood flows back strongly into the organ and limbs, improving overall circulation. The free arm adds to your firm foot foundation.

> **caution**
> Don't fold forward until your leg and foot are correctly positioned, or unnecessary pressure will be put on your knee, which could lead to injury. Do not progress any further through the sequences if this posture is not correct.

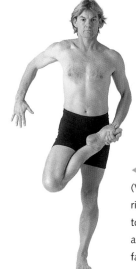

▲ 1 Exhaling
Stand with firm foundation in *Samasthitih* (*see p. 38*).

◀ 2 Inhaling
(Vinyasa 1) Without using your hands, raise your right knee and foot up along your central axis toward your chest. Keeping your foot on the central axis, open up your hip and allow your right knee to fall to the right side. Now, using your hands, support your right foot and take your thighbone well back to maximize the opening of your hips. Relax your calf muscle and bring your heel into your lower left abdomen above the pubic bone. Hold your foot in place with your left hand, extend out through your right arm, and begin to reach wide around behind your back.

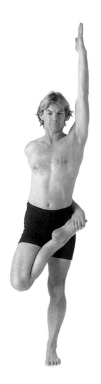

◀ 3 Still inhaling

(Vinyasa 1) Continue to reach around behind your back with your right hand until you can take hold of either your left elbow or wrist. Complete your binding by sliding your right hand down to hold your right foot. Now reach up with your left hand and gaze to nasagrai dristi.

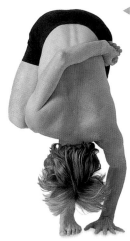

◀ 4 Exhaling (x 5 breaths)

(Vinyasa 2) Bend your right knee slightly to access ankle flexion and hip rotation. Keep your hips level and fold forward to place your left hand on to the mat beside your left foot. Pull up on your kneecap and thigh to straighten your left leg. Share the foundation between your hand and foot to help avoid hyperextending the knee joint of the standing leg. Gaze to nasagrai dristi and breathe deeply for five full breaths.

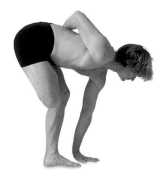

▲ 5 Inhaling–Exhaling

(Vinyasa 3) Inhale as you press strongly through your right hand, extend forward through your torso, and look up to the horizon. As you exhale, hold this position to ensure firm bandha application. At the end of your exhalation, transfer your body weight from your hand into you standing leg and bend your knee.

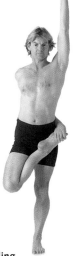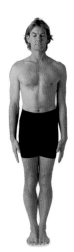

▲ 6–7 Inhaling–Exhaling

(Vinyasa 4) Inhaling, slowly stand through your left leg, reach up with your left arm and look to nasagrai dristi. As you exhale (vinyasa 5), release your foot and lower your right leg, returning to *Samasthitih*. For the left side vinyasas, repeat the preceding steps, reversing lefts and rights.

Sequence 1:

Fierce Posture
Utkatasana

Utkata means "fierce" or "powerful". It is here that we return to *Surya Namaskara* (*see pp. 24–5*) for the sequence into and out of the asana known as the Fierce Posture. *Utkatasana* marks the beginning of what is called the "Warrior Sequence". This pose powerfully stretches your Achilles tendon and shins as you sit down deeply into an imaginary seat. Your arms reach upward with force as your hands press firmly together in upward prayer. At the same time, your sacrum and tailbone pull down to lengthen your spine.

◀ **1–7 Inhaling–Exhaling**
From *Samasthitih* (*see p. 38*), inhale and exhale as you flow through vinyasas 1–6 of *Surya Namaskara A* (*see pp. 24–5*), finishing on an exhalation in the Downward-facing Dog position. From here onward, this sequence will be called "vinyasa down" and regarded as a single step.

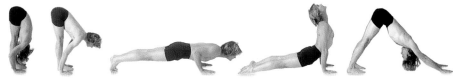

▼ **10 Exhaling**
Keeping your knees bent, bring your hands down and place them beside your feet, a shoulder-distance apart. Now look to a spot at the front of your mat and press your hands firmly into the mat.

◀ **8 Inhaling**
(Vinyasa 7) Look forward to a spot at the front of your mat and jump your feet together between your hands. Sit down into your heels, shins, and thighs. Tuck your tailbone down, lengthening the back of your neck, and begin to raise your arms to the sides.

▶ **9 Still inhaling**
(Vinyasa 7) Continue to look to the mat to lengthen and free your neck and shoulders. Raise your arms, rolling your shoulders down, bring your hands together and reach up in prayer. Look up to urdhva dristi, and breathe deeply for five full breaths.

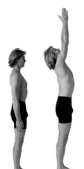

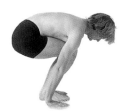
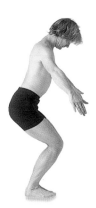

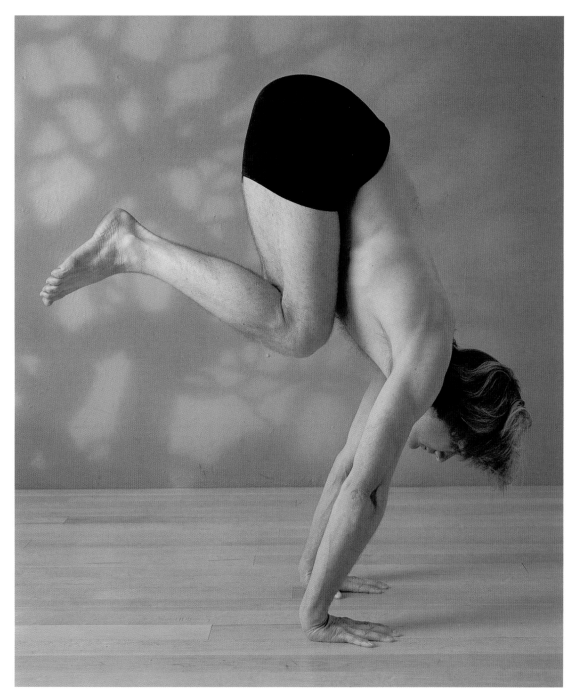

▲ **11 Inhaling**

(Vinyasa 8) Press further into the mat, bringing your shoulders well forward of your wrists. Using mula and uddiyana bandhas, lift up on to your hands. Keep your feet and knees tucked in and maintain balance for all of the inhalation. Exhaling, jump back to the 4th position of *Surya Namaskara* and then "vinyasa up" *Samasthitih*, as described on page 67, step 8.

Sequence 1:
Warrior Sequence
Virabhadrasana

Vira means "hero" and *Virabhadra* himself was created by the Hindu god Lord Shiva. Shiva pulled a lock from his matted hair, threw it to the ground, and a mighty warrior sprang forth to receive his orders. The Warrior Sequence is a powerful conclusion to the standing postures, taking you back to the beginning – *Surya Namaskara* (*see pp. 24–5*). This time, instead of flowing through the warrior pose, you hold for five deep breaths. You will experience being held between the power of stepping forward and the strength of stillness. Your arms, straight like a warrior's sword, are first held upward in the prayer position and then opened wide to the sides, opening the heart.

▼ **1 Vinyasa down**
(Vinyasas 1–6) Flow through this sequence of moves to Downward-facing Dog (*see p. 64*).

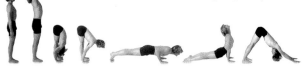

▶ **2 Inhaling (x 5 breaths)**
(Vinyasa 7) Inhaling, turn your left heel in to align with your right big toe, step forward with your right foot and place it between your hands, beside your right thumb. Raise your torso and square your hips forward by directing your right buttock back and the left side of your groin forward. Tuck your tailbone down and sit into your pelvis and right thigh until your knee is positioned over your right foot. Reach up with your arms, press your hands together, and look to urdhva dristi (*see p. 23*). Breathe deeply for five full breaths.

▼ **3 Inhaling**
(Vinyasa 8) Maintaining your upward prayer position, straighten your right leg. Turn your right foot in and your left foot out, turning your body to face the left side of your mat.

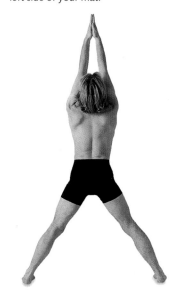

◀ 4 Inhaling (x 5 breaths)

(Vinyasa 8) Inhaling, turn your right foot in and your left foot out, and turn your body to face the back of the mat. Exhaling, bend your left leg 90°, bringing your knee over your left foot. Tuck your tailbone down and square your hips by directing your left buttock back and the right side of your groin forward. Draw your abdomen in to engage uddiyana and mula bandhas. Continue looking to urdhva dristi and breathe deeply for five full breaths.

▶ 5 Exhaling (x 5 breaths)

(Vinyasa 9) Exhaling, keep your left leg bent at a right angle. Bring your arms down to shoulder height (palms down), turning your right foot out to 90° and slightly lengthen your stance. Roll your right thigh up and turn your torso to the left of the mat. Draw your abdomen in, tuck your tailbone down, lengthen your spine, and look to hastagrai dristi. Breathe deeply for five full breaths.

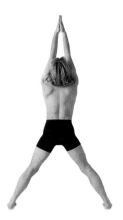

▲ 6 Inhaling

(Vinyasa 10) Repeat the instructions for step 3, reversing rights and lefts.

▶ 7 Exhaling–Inhaling

(Vinyasa 10) Turn your right foot out to face the front of the mat and bend your knee to 90°. Now repeat the instructions for step 5, reversing rights and lefts. Hold this position for five full breaths and on the last exhalation turn so that your torso is facing forward and place your hands down either side of your right foot. Inhaling, press firmly into your hands and then jump up and exhale.

▶ 8 Vinyasa up

To vinyasa up, flow through the concluding vinyasas of *Surya Namaskara A* (see pp. 24–5), finishing in *Samasthitih*.

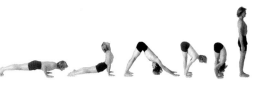

Sequence 2:
The Seated Sequence

In this phase of the practice session, we are now moving from a standing foundation to a seated one as we continue to weave asanas on to the thread of the breath. During both the entry into and exit out of the seated asanas, the benefits of Vinyasa (*see pp. 14–17*) can be more fully appreciated. As with the standing sequence, *Samasthitih* (*see p. 38*) is the neutral position that links the beginning and the end of each seated asana. By starting and returning to this standing, contemplative pose, it is possible to bring your body back to centre and more effectively to regulate your breath.

Starting from *Samasthitih*, there is a sequence of seven movements that lead us into the seated asana and a sequence of six movements that lead us out of the asana and back to *Samasthitih*. To simplify the instructions for this, the movements that lead us from standing in *Samasthitih* down to the seated asana are termed "vinyasa down" (*see p. 64*); the sequence of movements leading from the seated asana back to *Samasthitih* are termed "vinyasa up" (*see p. 67*); and where a pose is repeated on both sides – in other words, on the left and right sides – there is a "half vinyasa" between them composed of three movements. It is important to note, however, that there are poses that have a vinyasa specific to them and do not follow the general rule.

The traditional method of practice is termed "full vinyasa", but it is possible to practise an abbreviated form by substituting the full vinyasa (vinyasa up and vinyasa down) with the half vinyasa, thus jumping through to the seated position between each asana and between the right and left repetitions.

In the following sequences of seated postures, we are exploring new territory with regards to foundation. Here we are connecting to the ground directly through the pelvis, and no longer through the legs to the pelvis. Not only do we begin to explore this new relationship to the ground but we also begin to explore how we lift our body from the ground "up" and "back" every time we change sides or move to the next pose. This form of lifting is an intrinsic part of the practice, and it can take a long time to perfect.

For each of the seated asanas there is a lift and an appropriate transition out of the pose. As a beginner, these transitions will not be possible until your inner strength (bandhas) and external strength have been sufficiently developed.

Most of the seated asanas in Yoga Chikitsa (*see p. 15*) concentrate on forward bending, although periodically we have a semi-backbend to act as a counterpose to this. Shri K Pattabhi Jois makes it clear in his teachings that practitioners must develop forward bending for internal reasons before progressing to backbending. Although many people have naturally flexible spines, they do not necessarily have the internal strength to support backbending. It is here, in the seated postures, that we further cultivate the inner work (bandhas) begun in the standing asana.

OPPOSITE *This asana, called* Kukkutasana, *or Rooster (see pp. 104–5), demonstrates a combination of balance, poise, grace, and strength. It resembles a rooster in the way that the chest is puffed forward and the hands look like the feet of a bird. This is one of the few poses where mula bandha can be released.*

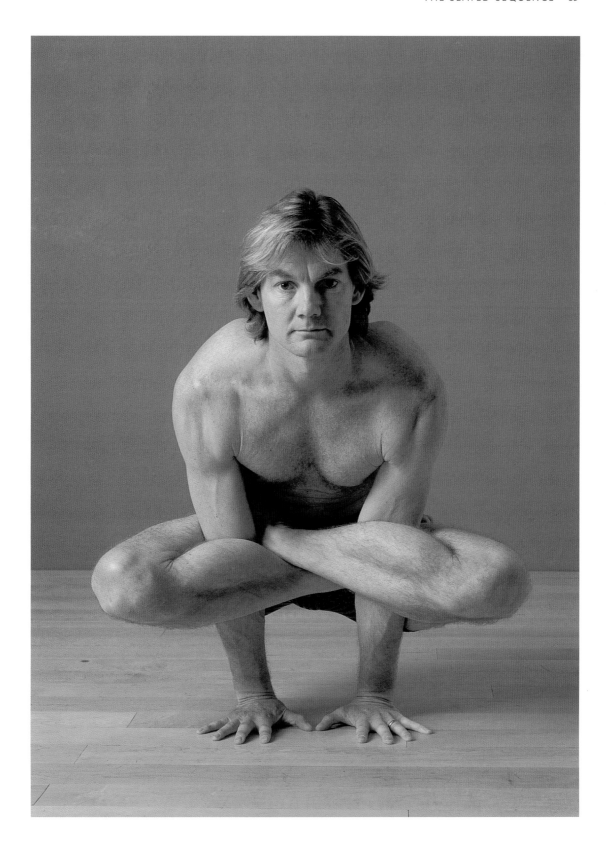

Sequence 2:

Jump Through

This sequence details the transition from Downward-facing Dog to Seated Staff (*Dandasana*), and demonstrates the most graceful aspects of "vinyasa down". Beginners often believe that they have to jump their whole body through their arms; in fact, it is only the legs. To better understand this transition, it can be described as "jump up to the point of balance, and then sit down". All of the techniques required to *float* your legs through your arms can be learned in *Surya Namaskara A*, or Sun Salute A (*see pp. 24–5*). If you pay attention to developing the strength and flexibility of your wrists in vinyasas 3 and 7 your hands will provide the necessary foundation to support your whole body. This sequence cultivates mula and uddiyana bandhas (*see pp. 21–3*), providing the inner strength needed to lift your body into flight.

> **tip**
> Lifting your head by the use of dristis, or looking places (see p. 23), helps to prevent your natural reflex to forward roll. Looking forward also accurately locates the correct landing spot.

◀ **1 Exhaling**

(Vinyasa 6) Move into Downward-facing Dog and look toward the nabi chakra dristi (*see p. 23*). Focus your internal gaze on the mula and uddiyana bandhas. Don't tense your lower abdomen – this inhibits the length and lifting effect of the next inhalation. Feet are parallel and aligned with your hips; hands a shoulder-width apart. Spread your fingers, middle fingers pointing forward. Avoid collapsing your shoulders as this will restrict your breath and reduce the necessary extension out of the shoulders needed as you move into the next position.

▶ **2 Still exhaling**

(Vinyasa 7) Exhaling further into the bandhas (*see pp. 21–3*), lift your head by changing the dristi from your navel to the space between your hands, and then on further to about 30cm (12in) in front of your hands (*see tip box*). Bring your shoulders forward and extend out of them, coming up on to your toes with knees bent. Rock back, ready to spring. Now start your next inhalation.

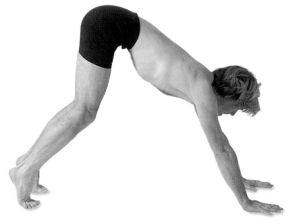

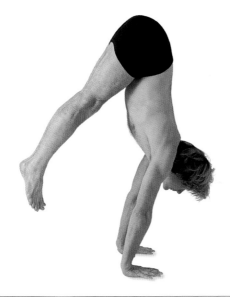

◄ **3 Inhaling**

Press firmly through your hands and spring up, as if jumping over an obstacle, bringing your feet together. The path of your buttocks is an upward arc, which shifts the foundation fully on to your hands, allowing your head, shoulders, and upper back to pivot well forward of your wrists. Now your body is in equilibrium, moving neither up nor down. Keep your eyes focused on the dristi forward of your hands while your hands and bandhas resist the landing.

▼ **4 Still inhaling**

Keep the lifting action in the legs and bandhas activated as you inhale. Flex further forward to bring your centre of balance well over your hands. While maintaining the lift from the shoulders, allow your legs to swing through the space between your arms, and then change the dristi to padhayoragrai (toes). By looking at your toes, it is easier to keep connected to your feet and your legs lifted.

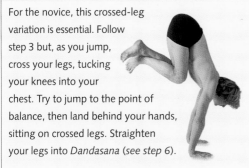

For the novice, this crossed-leg variation is essential. Follow step 3 but, as you jump, cross your legs, tucking your knees into your chest. Try to jump to the point of balance, then land behind your hands, sitting on crossed legs. Straighten your legs into *Dandasana* (see step 6).

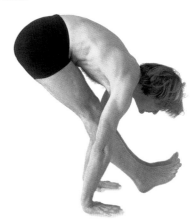

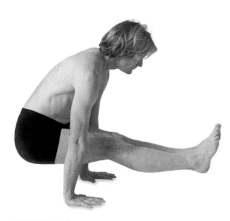

▲ **5 Still inhaling**

Gazing at the padhayoragrai (toes) dristi, resist the temptation to crash land on the mat. A controlled landing will further develop the strength in your arms and help to reinforce and cultivate the inner lift.

◄ **6 Exhaling**

Slowly rest your buttocks on the mat in *Dandasana*. Keep your hands pressing down until the end of the exhalation. Now draw the dristi in, moving it to the tip of your nose (nasagrai). Advanced students can aim to jump through and get into the ready position for the next asana all in one long inhalation.

Sequence 2:

Jump Back

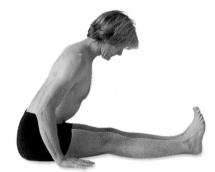

Technically, Jump Back is the reverse of Jump Through (*see pp. 70–1*), and this sequence of movements demonstrates the most graceful aspects of the "vinyasa up". This series details the correct lift required for the flowing transition out of the seated asanas. The Jump Back is advanced because, unlike the Jump Through, you do not benefit from the momentum created by the action of jumping to initiate the lift off the floor. To perform this successfully, the cultivation of mula and uddiyana bandhas (*see pp. 21–3*) must be present in order to resist the pull of gravity and overcome the inertia of your stationary body. The only way to master this lift is to practise the movement itself.

tip

Try adding in steps 1 and 2 of the sequence each time you finish the five breaths of a seated asana, before crossing your legs and rolling over your feet preparatory to jumping back to vinyasa 4 of *Surya Namaskara A.*

◄ **1 Exhaling**

Inhale as you sit tall in *Dandasana* (Seated Staff), shown on page 71, step 6. Then, exhaling, pivot from your hip joints, keeping your spine long and straight, and bring your shoulders forward of your hips and place your hands next to your thighs, midway between your knees and hips. Draw your abdomen in and look to your toes dristi.

▶ **2 Inhaling**

(Advanced) Press firmly into the floor with your hands while extending out of the shoulders, and lift your body, crossing your feet and drawing your knees toward your chest. (Intermediate) Develop a swinging pendulum effect by lifting your buttocks and cross legs forward and up, ready to swing back with the power of the next exhalation.

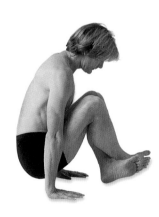

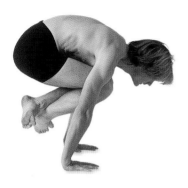

◀ **3 Inhaling–Exhaling**

(Advanced) Still lifting with the internal strength of the bandhas and power of the inhalation, pivot from your shoulder joints – swinging your buttocks and legs up and your head down. Allow your wrists to flex and keep your shoulders well forward so that the weight of your head counterbalances the weight of your buttocks and legs. (Intermediate) Exhale and swing your legs back and through your arms. You may have to touch the floor lightly with one or both of your feet.

▶ **4 Exhaling**

(Advanced) Using the momentum of movement and the directional control of uddiyana bandha, continue to lift your buttocks higher into the air. (Intermediate) Spring or jump with your feet to aid the lifting of your buttocks high into the air, until you reach a point of balance over your hands.

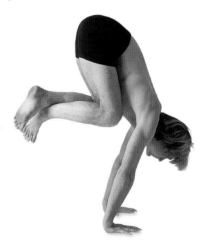

◀ **5 Still exhaling**

(Advanced, intermediate, beginner) Try to float on the exhalation as you maintain a forward direction with your upper body, while your legs begin to straighten ready for the landing. Try to keep a light pressure between your feet and knees while keeping your legs together as one unit. Now prepare to bend your elbows.

▶ **6 Still exhaling**

Bend your elbows 90° and extend forward with your chin. Completely straighten your legs, separating your feet so that they are a hip-distance apart, and land on the balls of your feet. Allow your feet to slide on the mat a little, adjusting to the full length of your legs and body. Keep the energy lifting up through your buttocks and legs and don't allow your upper torso to sink below the height of your elbows.

Sequence 2:

Seated Forward Bends
Paschimattanasana

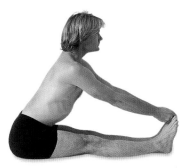 *Paschima* means "west" while "uttana" translates as "intense". In this asana, the word "west" refers to the back. Therefore, this asana is concerned with intensely stretching the entire back side of your body – from the heels to the crown of your head. Your torso extends from the hips, and you lengthen and draw in your abdomen as you fold forward over your legs. Uddiyana bandha (*see pp. 22–3*) is extremely important in all the forward bends, since it maintains length in the abdomen and helps to extend the spine evenly. *Paschimattanasana* prepares you for all the more complex variations of the forward bend that follow. Initially this pose can feel very difficult, but as you grow more familiar with it, it can become a place of solace and tranquillity.

> **tip**
> In step 4, opposite, don't pull yourself forward by the strength of your shoulders. Doing this will result in tension around your shoulders and neck, and block the free-flowing ujjayi breath (*see pp. 18–21*).

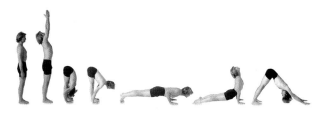

◀ **1 Vinyasa down**
(Vinyasas 1–6) Flow through this sequence of moves to Downward-facing Dog (*see p. 64*).

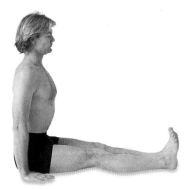

▲ **2 Inhaling (x 5 breaths)**
(Vinyasa 7) Jump through your arms and straighten your legs in *Dandasana* (Seated Staff) as described on page 71, step 6. Keep your hands pressed firmly into the mat to support and lengthen your spine. Draw in your abdomen, directing your breath up into your back and chest. Tuck in your chin slightly and gaze to the toes dristi. Breathe deeply for five full breaths.

▲ **3 Inhaling**
(Vinyasa 8) Maintaining the length in your spine, pivot forward from your hips to catch your big toes with the first two fingers of each hand. Engage uddiyana bandha and, inhaling, "open up" – lifting your chest away from your legs to create space and length from your pubic bone to sternum. Maintain the length in the neck and look to the third eye dristi. Now straighten your arms, legs, and back.

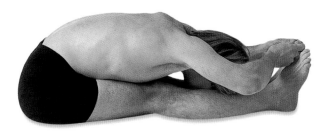

◀ 4 Exhaling (x 5 breaths)

(Vinyasa 9) Slightly release and bend your knees. Roll your pubic bone toward the mat, extend your torso over your legs, and take your chin to your shins. Pull up on your knees and thighs to straighten your legs. Look to the toes dristi and breathe deeply for five full breaths. Try to access the inner stretch from your bandha to the crown of your head. After the fifth exhalation, inhale and open up, as in step 2, in order to change to the hand variations below.

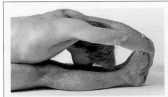 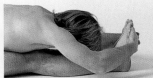 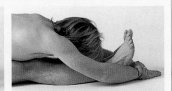

Exhaling, release your knees a little and change your hand position to the first variation (*above left*), hands over the top of your feet; hands holding the
sides of your feet (*above centre*); and holding your wrists beyond your feet (*above right*). Inhale and "open up", as in step 2, and pull up on your kneecaps
and thighs. Then, exhaling, fold over your legs into *Paschimattanasana*, following the instructions in step 4.

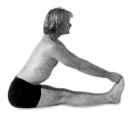 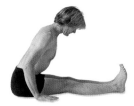 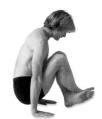

▲ 5–6–7 Inhaling–Exhaling–Inhaling

(Vinyasa 10) Inhale, open up, and look up, as in step 2. Keeping your shoulders forward of your hip joints, exhale and release your feet. Place your hands on the mat beside your thighs, as shown on page 72, step 1. (Vinyasa 11) Press strongly through your palms, cross and lift your legs off the mat, and draw your knees into your chest. Swing back and, exhaling, land in *Chatvari* (*see pp. 24–5*). To develop the inner body lift, you can repeat these three steps between each hand variation.

▼ 8 Vinyasa up

(Vinyasas 12–16) After completing the variations shown in detail above, flow through this sequence of moves to finish in *Samasthitih* (*see p. 67*).

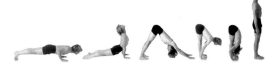

Sequence 2:

Seated Back Arch
Purvattanasana

Purva means "east" or "front" and *uttana* means "intense". This intense front body stretch is the necessary and the direct counterpose to the previous intense *Paschimattanasana* (*see pp. 74–5*). The principles of the primary series, or Yoga Chikitsa (*see p. 15*), are to align and purify the body, externally and internally, in order to prevent disease. Disease originates from an imbalance in organ functions, making it imperative to practise the asanas correctly and to link them together in a balanced and precise order. Here, at the beginning of the primary series, *Purtvattanasana* establishes the exact method of pose and counterpose. When an asana does not have a direct opposite stretch, then the folding forward and backward action of the connecting full or half vinyasa acts as the counterpose and so restores balance.

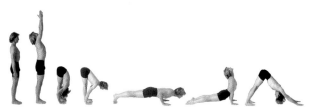

◀ **1 Vinyasa down**
Flow through this sequence of moves to Downward-facing Dog (*see p. 64*).

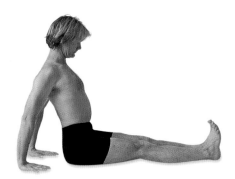

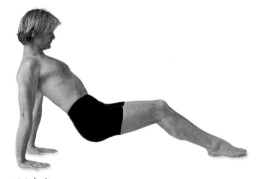

▲ **2 Exhaling**
From Downward-facing Dog, jump through your arms to Seated Staff (*Dandasana*). As you exhale, roll your shoulders back as you place your hands flat on the mat, a shoulder-distance apart and approximately 20cm (8in) behind your buttocks, fingers pointing back toward you. Draw your abdomen in, lift your heart region, and look to your toes dristi.

▲ **3 Inhaling**
(Vinyasa 8) Pressing through the palms of your hands, bend your knees slightly and put your weight on to your heels. Point through your toes and place the soles of your feet flat and firmly on to the mat. Continuing to look at your toes dristi while you lift your body off the mat will help you secure your foot foundation.

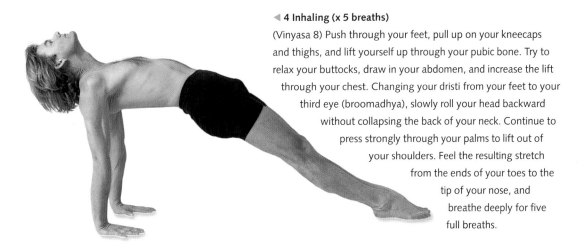

◀ 4 Inhaling (x 5 breaths)
(Vinyasa 8) Push through your feet, pull up on your kneecaps and thighs, and lift yourself up through your pubic bone. Try to relax your buttocks, draw in your abdomen, and increase the lift through your chest. Changing your dristi from your feet to your third eye (broomadhya), slowly roll your head backward without collapsing the back of your neck. Continue to press strongly through your palms to lift out of your shoulders. Feel the resulting stretch from the ends of your toes to the tip of your nose, and breathe deeply for five full breaths.

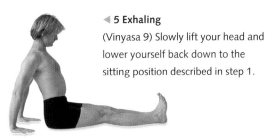

◀ 5 Exhaling
(Vinyasa 9) Slowly lift your head and lower yourself back down to the sitting position described in step 1.

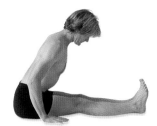

▲ 6 Still exhaling
(Vinyasa 9) Bend your torso forward and place your hands firmly on the mat beside your thighs, as described on page 74, step 1. Look to your toes dristi.

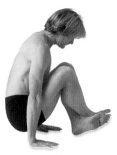

◀ 7 Inhaling
(vinyasa 10) Press strongly through your palms, cross and lift your legs off the mat, and draw your knees into your chest.
(Vinyasa 11) Swing back and, exhaling, land in *Chatvari*, as described on page 24.

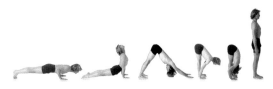

▲ 8 Vinyasa up
(Vinyasas 12–16) Flow through this sequence of moves to finish in *Samasthitih* (see p. 67).

Sequence 2:

Half-lotus Bound, Seated Forward Bend
Ardha Baddha Padma Paschimattanasana

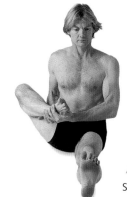

Ardha means "half", *baddha* translates as "bound", *padma* is "lotus", *paschima* means "west", and *uttana* is "intense". This is the seated variation of the intense, Half-lotus Bound, Standing Forward Bend (*see pp. 62–3*). Due to the seated foundation here, the effect of gravity intensifies the depth and pressure of the lotus heel into the liver and spleen. The full cleansing effects of this asana will be achieved only if the positioning of your heel is correct. Pay particular attention to optimizing your hip rotation to locate your heel in your lower abdomen, just above your pubic bone. The binding ensures that there is resistance against which your foot can flex, and this, in turn, presses your heel deeper into your organs.

◀ 1 Vinyasa down
(Vinyasas 1–6) Flow through this sequence of moves to Downward-facing Dog (*see p. 64*).

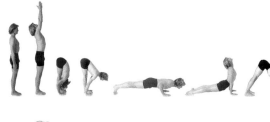

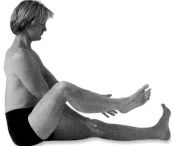

▲ 2 Inhaling
(Advanced) Jump through into *Dandasana* and, without using your hands, lift your right leg and draw your heel in toward your hands. Continue inhaling for the following steps, 3–6. (Intermediate) Until you cultivate a long, flowing inhalation, jump through to *Dandasana* on an inhalation and then, as you exhale, lift your right leg and draw your heel in toward your hands.

▲ 3 Still inhaling
Sit tall and support your right foot with your hands. Relax your thigh and buttocks. Now, leading with your leg and assisting with your hands, move your thighbone well back in order to maximize the opening of your hip. Relax your calf muscle and bring your lower leg across on the inside line of the knee joint. Do not force your knee.

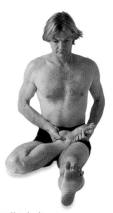 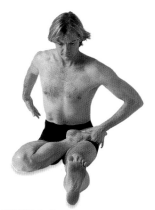 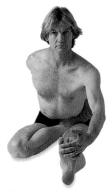

▲ 4 Still inhaling
Bring your right heel into your lower left abdomen, just above the pubic bone. Hold your right foot in place and roll your shinbone and knee down toward the mat.

▲ 5 Still inhaling
The correct heel placement will result in only your toes extending out beyond your waist. Hold your right foot in place with your left hand and extend out through your right arm to reach wide around behind your back.

▲ 6 Still inhaling
(Vinyasa 7) Continue to reach around behind your back to take hold of your right big toe. Now reach forward with your left hand and take hold of your left foot. Lift your chest away from your straight left leg until your left arm is straight. Square your shoulders and gaze to nasagrai dristi.

▶ 7 Exhaling (x 5 breaths)
(Vinyasa 8) Extending over your heel and maintaining the length in your spine, fold forward from your hips and take your chin toward the shin of your left leg. Flex the foot of your bound half-lotus to ensure deep pressure into the spleen, liver, and bowel. Gaze to padhayoragrai dristi (toes) and breathe deeply for five full breaths. Note that if you cannot bind your lotus foot, then don't fold down over your straight leg.

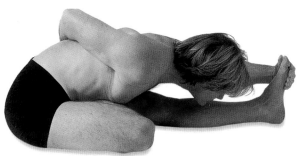

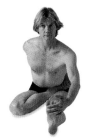

▲ 8–9 Inhaling
(Vinyasa 9) Inhale and open up your chest, as in step 6. Exhaling, release your binding, cross your legs, and place your hands on the mat forward of your hips. (Vinyasa 10) Inhale as you press firmly into the floor, lift and, exhaling, swing back to *Chatvari* (see p. 24).

▼10 Half vinyasa
(Vinyasas 11–13) Half vinyasa to the left side, jumping through again to step 2. From this point, repeat the following steps, changing the directions for rights and lefts. After completing the left side, vinyasa up (vinyasas 18–22) to *Samasthitih* (see p. 67).

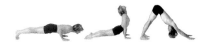

Sequence 2:

One Leg Folded Back
Tiriangmukhaikapada Paschimattanasana

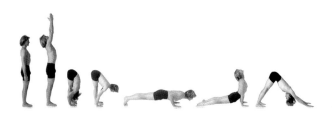

Tiriang means "transverse", *mukha* is "face", *ikapada* translates as "one foot" or "leg", *paschima* means "west", and *uttana* is "intense". When you place a leg into the Lotus, the lower half of the leg is folded inward on the inside line of the knee joint. This asana is the counterpose to the previous one (*see pp. 78–9*), and the lower leg here is folded transversely, facing back along the outside line of the knee joint. As a pair, *Ardha Baddha Padma Paschimattanasana* and *Tiriangmukhaikapada Paschimattanasana* facilitate the opening of the hip joints – first, the outward rotation of the hip and then, second, the inward rotation – preparing you for the deeper hip work required by the following asanas.

◀ **1 Vinyasa down**
(Vinyasas 1–6) Flow through this sequence of moves to Downward-facing Dog (*see p. 64*).

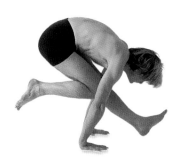

▲ **2 Inhaling**
(Vinyasa 7) From Downward-facing Dog, (advanced) jump into the air and bend your right leg backward from the knee. At the point of balance, keep the lift in order to bring your straight left leg through your arms. Keep looking to a spot on the mat in front of you and prepare to land on your right bent leg. (Intermediate) Jump through to *Dandasana*.

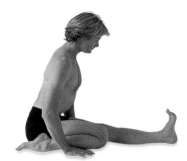

▲ **3 Still inhaling**
(Vinyasa 7) Lower yourself gently down on to the top of your right foot and position your buttocks squarely on the mat (advanced). The heel of your right foot is now adjacent to your right hip and your shinbone presses directly down into the mat. Flex your left foot and change your dristi to your toes. (Intermediate) Lean on to your left buttock and fold your right leg back.

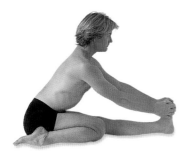

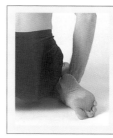

To ground both buttocks, it may be necessary to soften and roll your calf muscle on your folded leg out to the side. To do this, roll the flesh of your inside thigh up and tuck the flesh of your outer thigh down toward the mat.

▲ **4 Still inhaling**

(Vinyasa 7) Extend your spine out of your pelvis and reach forward with both hands to take hold of your left foot. Open up and lift your chest away from your straight left leg until your arms are straight. Now square your shoulders and sit down into your right buttock so that your hips are square. Draw in your abdomen and gaze to the third eye dristi.

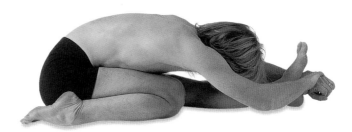

▲ **5 Exhaling (x 5 breaths)**

(Vinyasa 8) Maintaining the extension out of your pelvis, fold forward over your left leg. To avoid falling over on your straight leg side, sit further into your right folded leg at the same time as you extend out through your left buttock. Look to the foot dristi and breathe deeply for five full breaths.

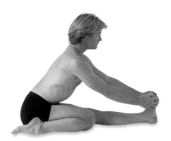

▲ **6–7 Inhaling–Exhaling**

(Vinyasa 9) Inhale and open up, as in step 4. Exhaling, keep your torso extending forward, release your hold, and place your hands on to the mat beside your thighs. (Vinyasa 10) Inhaling, keep your right leg bent and lift your body up off the mat. Fold your left leg and prepare to swing back to *Chatvari* (see pp. 24–5).

▶ **8 Half vinyasa**

(Vinyasas 11–13) Half vinyasa to the left side, jumping through again to step 2. From this point, repeat the following steps, changing the directions for rights and lefts. After completing the left side, vinyasa up (vinyasas 18–22) to *Samasthitih* (see p. 67).

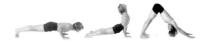

Sequence 2:
Head of the Knee A
Janu Sirsasana A

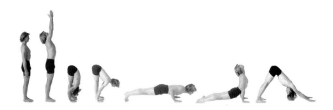 *Janu* means "knee" and *sirsa* translates as "head". *Janu Sirsasana A* is the first of three hip angles with heel variations. In this version, your bent knee is set at about a 90–95° angle to your straight leg, and your heel is placed against your perineum. This is the first seated asana to introduce a slight twist in the spine and you must take care to engage the bandhas to align correctly and protect your lower back (*see pp. 21–3*). The heat and pressure of the heel against your perineum stimulates the functions of the pancreas in men. This asana is also believed to help alleviate the symptoms of cystitis.

◀ **1 Vinyasa down**
(Vinyasas 1–6) Flow through this sequence of moves to Downward-facing Dog (*see p. 64*).

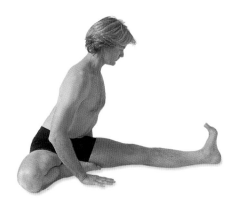

▲ **2 Inhaling**
(Vinyasa 7) From Downward-facing Dog, jump up and fold your right leg in (advanced). At the point of balance, keep the lift going to bring your straight left leg through your arms. Land lightly on the mat, positioning your heel against your perineum and your knee out to the right side at 90–95°. (Intermediate) Jump through to *Dandasana* and fold your right heel in to press against your perineum.

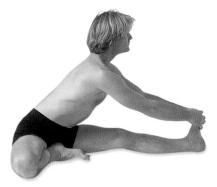

▲ **3 Still inhaling**
(Vinyasa 7) Take hold of your left foot and lift your chest away from your straight left leg until your arms are straight. Now square your shoulders and sit down into your buttocks. To correct the twisting action of your spine, pull back on your left buttock and roll your right hip forward. Engage your bandhas and centre your navel on the inside line of your straight leg. Gaze to the third eye.

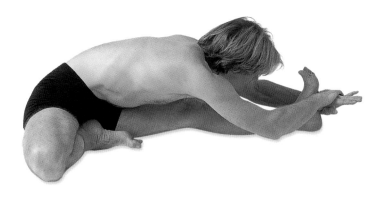

◀ **4 Exhaling (x 5 breaths)**

(Vinyasa 8) Maintaining the extension out of your pelvis, equalize the length from your hip joint to armpit on both sides. Bringing your navel forward to your thigh, bend your elbows and fold your torso over your left leg. Focus on your mula bandha to root down through your buttocks. Continue to draw in the uddiyana bandha to maintain the length and strength in your lower back. Look to padhayoragrai (foot) dristi and breathe deeply for five full breaths.

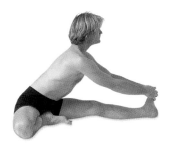
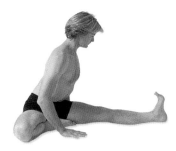
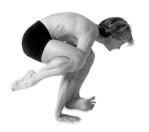

▲ **5–6–7 Inhaling–Exhaling–Inhaling**

(Vinyasa 9) Inhale and "open up" by lifting your chest away from your straight leg, as in step 3, and take hold of your left foot with both hands. Exhaling, keep your shoulders well forward of your hips, release your hold, and place your left hand on the mat beside your left thigh and your right hand on to the mat just forward of your right shin. (Vinyasa 10) Inhaling, lift your body up off the mat and slide your right shin up the back of your right arm. Fold your left leg and prepare to swing back to *Chatvari* position (*see pp. 24–5*).

▶ **8 Half vinyasa**

(Vinyasas 11–13) Half vinyasa to the left side, jumping through again to step 2. From this point, repeat the following steps, changing the directions for rights and lefts. After completing the left side, vinyasa up (vinyasas 18–22) to *Samasthitih* (*see p. 67*).

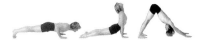

Sequence 2:
Head of the Knee B
Janu Sirsasana B

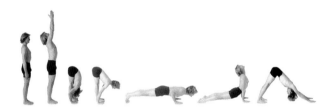

In *Janu Sirsana B*, the second variation, the head of your bent knee is set at an angle of 85° to your straight leg, and your heel is placed directly under your anus. Sitting the anus directly on to your heel helps to reinforce the physical connection to mula bandha. As in the first sequence of this series (*see pp. 82–3*), *Janu Sirsasana B* is also of particular benefit to men in stimulating and tonifying the urinary system. By sitting on your heel you stretch and strengthen your ankle joint, and it is also a preparatory stretch before moving on to the following variation.

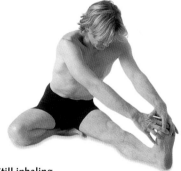

◀ **1 Vinyasa down**
(Vinyasas 1–6) Flow through this sequence of moves to Downward-facing Dog (*see p. 64*).

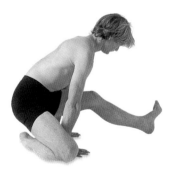

▲ **2 Inhaling**
(Vinyasa 7) From Downward-facing Dog jump up and fold your right leg in (advanced). At the point of balance, keep the "lift" going to bring your straight left leg through your arms. As you lower yourself down, position your heel so that it aligns with your anus, and then sit fully down on to your heel. (Intermediate) Jump through to *Dandasana*. Fold your right heel in toward your perineum, push through your hands and lift your body up. Move forward to sit your anus on to your heel.

▲ **3 Still inhaling**
(Vinyasa 7) Position your knee at an angle of 85° to your straight leg and then take hold of your left foot and open up your chest by lifting it away from your straight leg until your arms are at full stretch. Square your shoulders. Flex your right foot to ensure your anus engages with your heel and focus on mula bandha. The instep of your right foot should run along the underside of your left thigh. Centre your navel on the inside line of your straight leg and gaze to your third eye dristi.

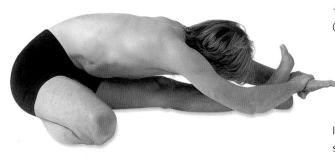

◀ 4 Exhaling (x 5 breaths)

(Vinyasa 8) Maintaining the extension out of your pelvis, equalize the length from your hip joint to armpit on both sides. Bend forward, bringing your navel to your thigh, bend your elbows, and fold your torso over your left leg. Pull up on your left kneecap and thigh and draw up on your anal sphincters to maintain the contact with your heel. Continue to draw in uddiyana bandha to maintain the length and strength in your lower back. Look to the foot dristi and breathe deeply for five full breaths.

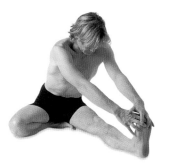
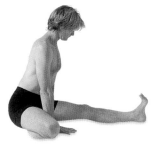
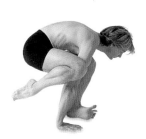

▲ 5–6–7 Inhaling–Exhaling–Inhaling

(Vinyasa 9) Inhale as you open up your chest, as in step 3, and take hold of your left foot with both hands. Exhaling, keeping your shoulders well forward of your hips, release the hold on your foot, and place your left hand on the mat beside your left thigh and your right hand on to the mat just forward of your right shin. (Vinyasa 10) Inhaling, lift your body up off the mat, sliding your right shin up the back of your right arm. Fold your left leg and prepare to swing back to *Chatvari* (see pp. 24–5).

▶ 8 Half vinyasa

(Vinyasas 11–13) Half vinyasa to the left side, jumping through again to step 2. From this point, repeat the following steps, changing the directions for rights and lefts. After completing the left side, vinyasa up (vinyasas 18–22) to *Samasthitih* (see p. 67).

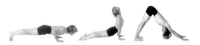

Sequence 2:

Head of the Knee C
Janu Sirsasana C

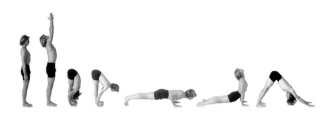
In *Janu Sirsana C*, the third variation, the head of the bent knee is set at an angle of 45° to the straight leg and your heel is aligned with your navel. The heat and pressure from the heel as you fold forward is of particular benefit to women, as the energy channels that stimulate the pancreas are located here, just below the navel. This asana is also beneficial for the female reproductive system, but take note that it should not be practised if you are pregnant. Correct placement of the heel in this asana is dependent on the range of hip rotation you have and the length of your Achilles tendon, and so it may take time to achieve. Take care with this asana to protect your knees.

caution
Do not practise this asana if you are pregnant.

◀ **1 Vinyasa down**
(Vinyasas 1–6) Flow through this sequence of moves to Downward-facing Dog (*see p. 64*).

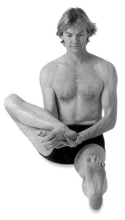

▲ **2 Inhaling**
(Vinyasa 7) From Downward-facing Dog jump through your arms to *Dandasana*, bend your right leg, and hold your right heel in your left hand. Now reach through the loop created and, with your right hand, take hold of your right toes. It is important to reach over your toes folding them back. Flex your right foot, extending out through your heel to stretch your Achilles tendon.

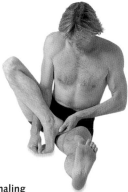

▲ **3 Still inhaling**
(Vinyasa 7) Lean on to your left buttock and release the flexion in your right foot. Turn your right toes down toward the mat at the same time as you place the ball of your foot on to the mat at 45° to your straight leg. Using your left hand, lift the heel of your right foot to a vertical position.

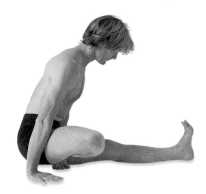

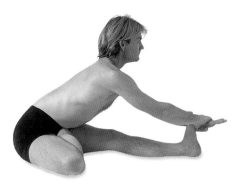

▲ **4 Still inhaling**
(Vinyasa 7) Slide your right hand out from under your right toes and place both hands down on the mat either side of your buttocks. Press strongly through your hands and lift your buttocks off the floor. Position your pelvis forward to bring your heel vertical and in line with your navel.

▲ **5 Still inhaling**
(Vinyasa 7) Sit your buttocks on the mat, roll your right thigh forward and bring your knee down to the mat at 45° to your straight leg. Reach forward, taking hold of your left foot, and "open up". Position your navel over your heel as you engage uddiyana bandha. Lift your chest away from your straight left leg until your arms are straight, and then square your shoulders. Look to your third eye dristi.

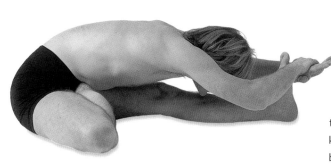

◀ **6 Exhaling (x 5 breaths)**
(Vinyasa 8) Bend your elbows and fold over your right heel to bring your chin to your left shin. Feel the deep pressure of your heel against your lower abdomen and navel. Maintain the length between your pubic bone and sternum as you extend your torso along your left leg. Pull up on your left kneecap and thigh. Look to the foot dristi and breathe deeply for five full breaths.

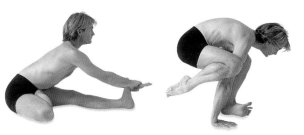

▲ **7–8 Inhaling–Exhaling–Inhaling**
(Vinyasa 9) Inhale and "open up", as described in step 5. Exhaling, keeping your shoulders well forward of your hips, release your hold and place your left hand on the mat beside your left thigh and your right hand on the mat just forward of your right shin. (Vinyasa 10) Inhaling, lift your body up off the mat and slide your right shin up the back of your right arm. Fold your left leg and prepare to swing back to *Chatvari* position (see pp. 24–5).

▼ **9 Half vinyasa**
(Vinyasas 11–13) Half vinyasa to the left side, jumping through again to step 2. From this point, repeat the following steps, changing the directions for rights and lefts. After completing the left side, vinyasa up (vinyasas 18–22) to *Samasthitih* (see p. 67).

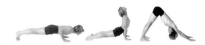

Sequence 2:

Sage Marichy, Son of Brahma A
Marichyasana A

In Hindu mythology, God Brahma is the creator of all. The asana demonstrated here is dedicated to Brahma's son, Marichy. Marichy was a great sage and the grandfather of Surya, the Sun God, whom we salute at the very beginning of practice – *Surya Namasakara*, or Sun Salutes (*see pp. 24–7*). It is believed that Marichy discovered this asana – one of eight variations, the first four of which are related to Yoga Chikitsa, the primary series, concerning body purification. The four variations – A, B, C, and D – are beneficial to the digestive system, clearing flatulence, indigestion, and constipation and improving digestive power generally. For women, these asanas are additionally beneficial for the reproductive system.

tip

The arm you use to bind around your bent knee is crucial. Try to extend your arms out of your shoulder joints in order to obtain maximum length, and so deepen the binding process.

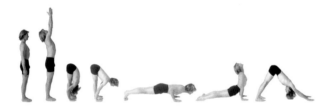

◀ **1 Vinyasa down**
(Vinyasas 1–6) Flow through this sequence of moves to Downward-facing Dog (*see p. 64*).

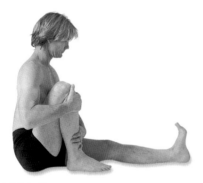

▲ **2 Inhaling**
(Vinyasa 7) From Downward-facing Dog, jump through to *Dandasana* and bend your right leg. Place your foot on the mat just in front of your right buttock, aligning your outer ankle with the outer face of your right hip joint. Flex your left foot back and sit tall through your spine and prepare to bind.

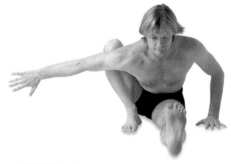

▲ **3 Still inhaling**
(Vinyasa 7) Place your left hand on the mat to the left side and, leaning into this additional foundation, push with your hand to fold your torso forward, past the inside of your right thigh. Fold from your hips, as in the Seated Forward Bends (*see pp. 74–5*). Now, extending out of your right shoulder, reach forward with your right arm and around your right shin.

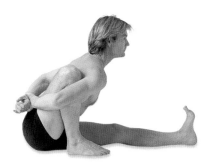

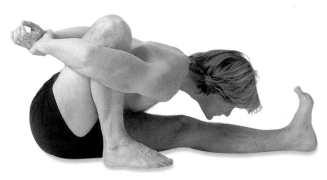

▲ 4 Still inhaling

(vinyasa 7) Roll your shoulder forward and fold your arm up behind your back. Transfer your weight to your right foot. Maximize the length of your left arm and bend it up behind your back. Hold your left wrist with your right hand and bring your left shoulder forward.

▲ 5 Exhaling (x 5 breaths)

(Vinyasa 8) Square your shoulders and press your bound right arm back. Tighten the binding and use the opposing forces between knee and arms to lever your torso down to touch your chin to your shin. Draw in uddiyana bandha, directing your breath to your chest and back, look to the foot dristi, and breathe deeply for five full breaths.

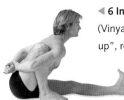

◀ 6 Inhaling

(Vinyasa 9) Inhale and "open up", returning to the position described in step 4.

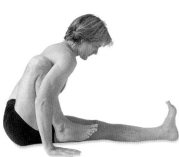

▲ 7 Exhaling

Keeping the opposing forces between your right armpit and right shin, release the binding and place your hands down on the mat. Lift your right foot off the mat and fix your gaze to your left foot.

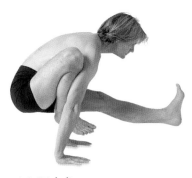

▲ 8–9 Inhaling

(Vinyasa 10) Press your right knee hard into the back of your right arm, engage your bandhas, tip your torso forward, and lift your left leg off the mat. Fold your left leg and look to a spot on the mat as you swing your legs through your arms, preparing to land in *Chatvari* (see p. 24).

▶ 10 Half vinyasa

(Vinyasas 11–13) Half vinyasa to the left side, jumping through again to step 2. From this point, repeat the following steps, changing the directions for rights and lefts. After completing the left side, vinyasa up (vinyasas 18–22) to *Samasthitih* (see p. 67).

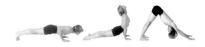

Sequence 2:

Sage Marichy, Son of Brahma B
Marichyasana B

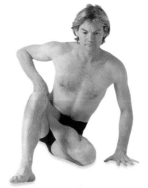

In *Marichyasana B*, the second variation, your straight leg is folded into the lotus position. Capturing your foot within the binding of your bent leg intensifies the depth and benefits of this asana. For women, the uterus benefits from being deeply massaged by your heel pressing into your lower abdomen. And if you normally experience painful periods, practising this asana may, in time, strengthen the uterus and improve menstrual function. The strengthening effect on the uterus may also help to reduce the risk of miscarriage. You should not practise this asana during menstruation. However, practising this asana habitually when you are not menstruating may lessen any pain associated with your monthly cycle.

> **caution**
>
> Note that because of this asana's effect on the uterus, women should discontinue performing this sequence after the second month of pregnancy.

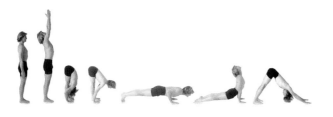

◀ **1 Vinyasa down**
(Vinyasas 1–6) Flow through this sequence of moves to Downward-facing Dog (*see p. 64*).

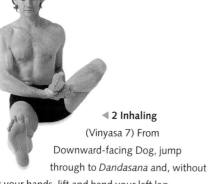

◀ **2 Inhaling**
(Vinyasa 7) From Downward-facing Dog, jump through to *Dandasana* and, without using your hands, lift and bend your left leg. Supporting your foot with your hands, relax your buttocks and thigh. Now, leading with your left leg, move your thighbone well back in order to maximize the opening of your hips.

◀ **3 Still inhaling**
(Vinyasa 7) Relax your left calf muscle and bring your left heel in to your lower right abdomen, just above the pubic bone. Holding your left foot in place with your right hand, place your left hand on the mat to your left. Lean into your left thigh to create a new foundation of thigh and hand. Bend your right leg and place your right foot on the mat just in front of your right buttock, aligning the outer face of your ankle with the outer face of your right hip joint.

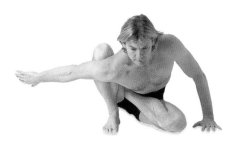

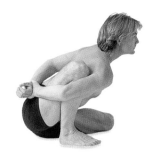

◀ 5 Still inhaling

(Vinyasa 7) Fold your arm up behind your back and transfer your weight on to your right foot. Extend out of your shoulder joint and bend your left arm up behind your back to meet your right hand. Hold your left wrist with your right hand. Bring your left shoulder forward and "open up".

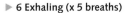

▲ 4 Still inhaling

(Vinyasa 7) Extend your torso over your left heel and reach beyond the inside of your right thigh with your right arm. Extending out of your shoulder, reach around your right shin. Your heel must be in your lower abdomen, with only the toes extending beyond your right thigh.

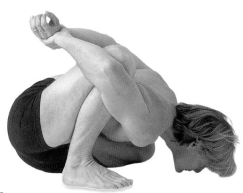

▶ 6 Exhaling (x 5 breaths)

(Vinyasa 8) Press your bound right arm back against your right shin and centre your chest between your left bent knee and right foot. Tighten your binding and lever your torso down and touch the mat with your chin. Your heel should press into uddiyana bandha. Look to nasagrai dristi and breathe deeply for five full breaths.

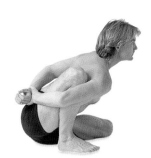

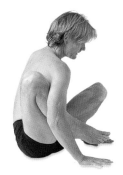

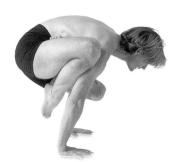

▲ 7 Inhaling

(Vinyasa 9) Inhale and "open up", returning to the position described in step 5.

▲ 8–9 Exhaling–Inhaling

Exhaling, release your binding and rock on your buttocks with your hands on the mat. Keep the pressure of your right shin into the back of your armpit. (Vinyasa 10) Inhaling, press your right knee into

the back of your right arm, engage the bandhas, tip forward, and lift up on to your hands. Look at a spot in front of the mat and prepare to swing back to *Chatvari* (see p. 24).

▶ 10 Half vinyasa

(Vinyasas 11–13) Half vinyasa to the left side, jumping through again to step 2. From this point, repeat the following steps, changing the directions for rights and lefts. After completing the left side, vinyasa up (vinyasas 18–22) to *Samasthitih* (see p. 67).

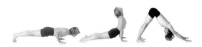

Sequence 2:

Sage Marichy, Son of Brahma C
Marichyasana C

In *Marichyasana C*, the third variation, your leg and pelvic foundation is the same as in *Marichyasana A* (*see pp. 88–9*), but instead of binding your bent leg with the arm of the same side, you bind with the opposite arm. This adds a rotating element to the posture, which has the effect of additionally massaging your lower abdomen and organs. This asana is also of benefit to your entire spine, since the rotation helps to create length and flexibility. The binding action restricts the lift of your ribcage and the expansion of the lung on the bound side, and in this way your ribcage on the opposite side develops greater expansion in order to achieve full inhalation. However, don't lean back and rotate through the lumbar spine before binding or you will place your intervertebral discs under too much pressure.

tip
Spinal rotation does not involve twisting from the pelvis. The binding works to sit you forward into a square pelvic foundation. You then lengthen out of the lumbar spine and rotate only in the thoracic spine.

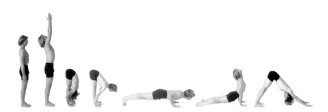

◀ **1 Vinyasa down**
(Vinyasas 1–6) Flow through this sequence of moves to Downward-facing Dog (*see p. 64*).

caution
Because this asana compresses the entire abdomen and uterus, pregnant women must not practise it.

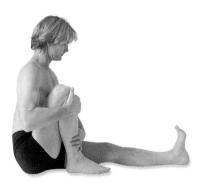

▲ **2 Inhaling**
(Vinyasa 7) From Downward-facing Dog, jump through to *Dandasana* and bend your right leg. Place your foot on the mat, just in front of your right buttock, aligning the outer ankle with your outer right hip joint. Flex your left foot back and sit tall through your spine and prepare to bind.

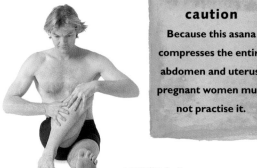

◀ **3 Still inhaling**
(Vinyasa 7) Place your right hand on the outside of your bent right leg. Turn your right foot in slightly, toward your left leg. Allow your right buttock to lift off the mat as you push your bent leg across your centre line to your left side.

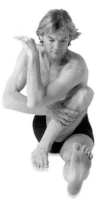

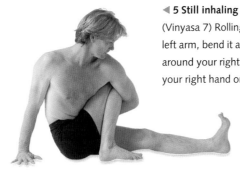

◀ 5 Still inhaling

(Vinyasa 7) Rolling your shoulder, rotate your left arm, bend it at the elbow, and feed it back around your right shin. You might need to place your right hand on the mat behind you to help to negotiate the binding, but do not lean back or initiate the spinal twist yet. Stay sitting forward and look to the front of your mat.

▲ 4 Still inhaling

(Vinyasa 7) Hold your bent right leg over to the left side and flex your torso to the right. Bend your left arm and, leading with the point of your elbow, fold forward to negotiate past your right bent leg. Try to fold forward until your left armpit touches your right thigh.

◀ 6 Inhaling (x 5 breaths)

(Vinyasa 7) Maintain your forward foundation and complete your binding – left hand holding your right wrist. Sit into your right foot and left leg. Work your right buttock toward the mat and sit tall from your pelvis. Leading with your sternum, rotate through the thoracic spine and look over your right shoulder to parsva dristi. Breathe deeply for five full breaths.

▶ 7– 8–9 Exhaling–Inhaling

Exhaling, release your binding, swing back to your centre, and place your hands on the mat, as shown on page 89, step 7. (Vinyasa 8) Press your right knee firmly into the back of your right arm, engage your bandhas, tip your torso forward, and lift your left leg off the mat. Now fold your left leg and look to a spot forward of the mat as you swing your legs through your arms and prepare to land in *Chatvari* (see p. 24).

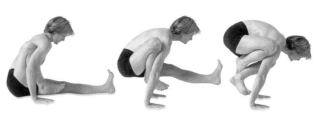

▶ 10 Half vinyasa

(Vinyasas 9–11) Half vinyasa to the left side, jumping through again to step 2. From this point, repeat the following steps, changing the directions for rights and lefts. After completing the left side, vinyasa up (vinyasas 14–18) to *Samasthitih* (see p. 67).

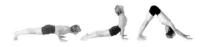

Sequence 2:

Sage Marichy, Son of Brahma D
Marichyasana D

In this sequence, the fourth variation, you incorporate the legwork seen in *Marichyasana B* and combine it with the twisting action of *Marichyasana C*. The result is an advanced asana and it shares the benefits of the three variations you have already seen. This is the most difficult asana up to this point in the primary series and is an excellent indicator of the level of expertise you have achieved. If, for example, you cannot perform this asana, then do not progress beyond this point. It is important to develop the required opening in your hips and ankles before you attempt any of the following asanas.

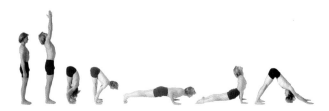

◀ **1 Vinyasa down**
(Vinyasas 1–6) Flow through this sequence of moves to Downward-facing Dog (*see p. 64*).

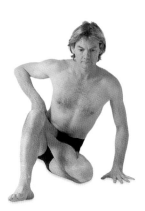

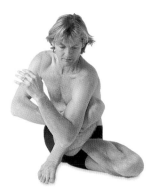

▲ **2 Inhaling**
(Vinyasa 7) From Downward-facing Dog, jump through to *Dandasana*, fold your left leg into the lotus, lean your thigh to the mat, and place your left hand down on the mat. Now bend your right leg and draw it in toward your right buttock. Align your outer ankle and outer right hip joint. Only the toes of your left foot should extend beyond your thigh. Make sure foot placement is correct – don't draw your foot too far over.

▲ **3 Still inhaling**
(Vinyasa 7) Place your right hand on the outside of your bent right leg. Turn your right foot in slightly. Push your bent leg diagonally across your centre line, and past your lotus foot. Hold your bent right leg over to the left side and flex your torso to the right. Bend your left arm and, leading with the point of your elbow, take your armpit down to make contact with your right bent leg.

▶ **4 Still inhaling**

(Vinyasa 7) Rolling your shoulder, rotate your left arm, bending it at the elbow, and feed it back around your right shin. You might need to place your right hand on the mat behind you to help to facilitate the binding. Don't lean back or initiate the spinal twist yet. Stay sitting forward and look to the front of the mat.

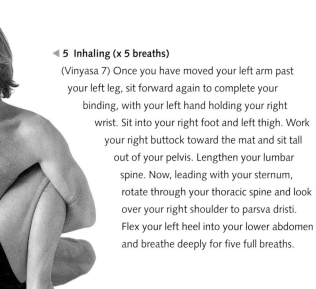

◀ **5 Inhaling (x 5 breaths)**

(Vinyasa 7) Once you have moved your left arm past your left leg, sit forward again to complete your binding, with your left hand holding your right wrist. Sit into your right foot and left thigh. Work your right buttock toward the mat and sit tall out of your pelvis. Lengthen your lumbar spine. Now, leading with your sternum, rotate through your thoracic spine and look over your right shoulder to parsva dristi. Flex your left heel into your lower abdomen and breathe deeply for five full breaths.

▶ **6–7 Exhaling–Inhaling**

Exhaling, release your binding, and recentre your body. Place your hands on the mat. (Vinyasa 8) Keeping the pressure of your right shin in the back of your right armpit, engage your bandhas. Inhaling, tip forward, lift up, and balance on your hands. To stop yourself falling forward, lift your head and look to a spot forward of the mat and prepare to land in *Chatvari* (see p. 24).

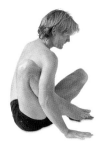
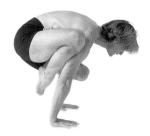

▶ **8 Half vinyasa**

(Vinyasas 9–11) Half vinyasa to the left side, jumping through again to step 2. From this point, repeat the following steps, changing the directions for rights and lefts. After completing the left side, vinyasa up (vinyasas 14–18) to *Samasthitih* (see p. 67).

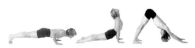

Sequence 2:
The Boat
Navasana

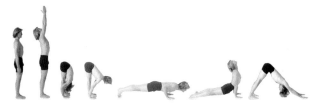

Nava means "boat" and this asana gets its name because the posture resembles the V-shaped keel of a boat. The main benefit of this asana is that it strengthens the spinal region. If your inner body is not strong and you have not developed the cultivation of bandhas by this stage of the practice, then *Navasana* can be deceptively difficult to perform correctly. To stay "afloat", the angle of your legs and back must be such that your toes and eyes are at the same height. Strong bandha control is necessary to maintain a straight spine and legs. The unseen energy harnessed by the bandhas is dynamically demonstrated as you lift your entire body gracefully through the space between your arms, up into a handstand, and then back down again – all without any part of your body or legs touching the floor.

◀ 1 Vinyasa down
(Vinyasas 1–6) Flow through this sequence of moves to Downward-facing Dog (*see p. 64*).

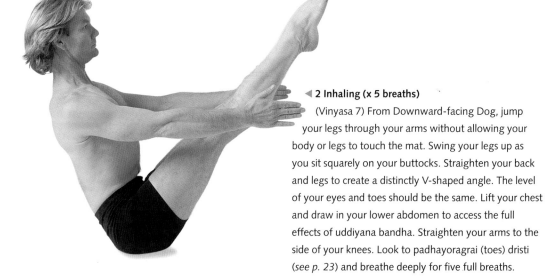

◀ 2 Inhaling (x 5 breaths)
(Vinyasa 7) From Downward-facing Dog, jump your legs through your arms without allowing your body or legs to touch the mat. Swing your legs up as you sit squarely on your buttocks. Straighten your back and legs to create a distinctly V-shaped angle. The level of your eyes and toes should be the same. Lift your chest and draw in your lower abdomen to access the full effects of uddiyana bandha. Straighten your arms to the side of your knees. Look to padhayoragrai (toes) dristi (*see p. 23*) and breathe deeply for five full breaths.

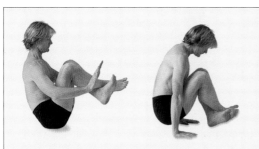

The alternative to the straight-leg lift is to cross your legs, without touching the floor, and draw them into your chest as you exhale. Rock forward into your hands, pressing firmly through your palms, and use the strength in your arms to lift your body off the floor. Keep your legs tucked in and resist the temptation to touch the mat with your feet.

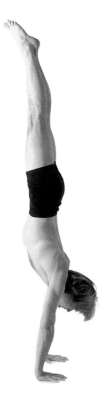

◀ 3 Exhaling
Maintaining the lift in your legs, place your hands on the mat just forward of your hips. Draw your abdomen in further and fully engage both mula and uddiyana bandhas. Drop your gaze downward and slightly shorten the front side of your body. Direct your internally harnessed energy firmly down through your palms into the mat.

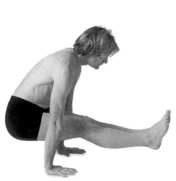

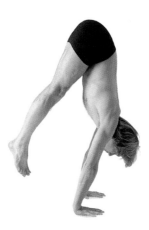

▲ 4–5–6 Inhaling–Exhaling
Pivot your shoulders forward of your wrists and, drawing up with uddiyana bandha, lift yourself. Engage your quadriceps and draw your legs back through your arms. Now, as you lower your head your buttocks rise. Continue up into a handstand. Exhaling, pivot from the hips and lower your legs through your arms. Land on your buttocks, raising your legs and arms into the Boat for five deep breaths. Repeat this sequence another four times, finally lowering yourself into *Chatvari* (see p. 24).

▼ 7 Vinyasa up
(Vinyasas 9–13) After completing the last handstand, flow through this sequence of moves to finish in *Samasthitih* (see p. 67).

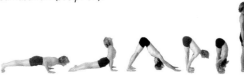

Sequence 2:
Arm Pressure Posture
Bhujapidasana

Bhuja means "arm" or "shoulder" and *pida* translates as "pressure". This is the first asana in which your body is supported entirely on the foundation formed by your arms and hands. Again, the internal energy harnessed by the bandhas is dynamically demonstrated through the transition into and out of this asana. Until the strength of your inner lift is developed, it will be necessary to jump to your feet and then to sit down on your arms. When the inner lift has been developed sufficiently, the aim is to jump into the final position in one movement. From the initial balancing position you require further strength and control to extend your chin forward to the mat. The stretch imparted to your esophagus is cleansing and purifying.

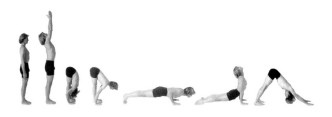

◀ **1 Vinyasa down**
(Vinyasas 1–6) Flow through this sequence of moves to Downward-facing Dog (*see p. 64*).

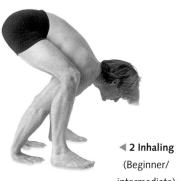

◀ **2 Inhaling**
(Beginner/ intermediate) From Downward-facing Dog, jump up into the air until you reach the point of balance. But instead of jumping through your arms, as you have now done many times in the practice, jump your legs around the outside of your arms and land on your feet.

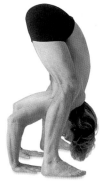

◀ **3 Still inhaling**
(Beginner) Transfer the weight of your body from your feet to your hands and, bending at the elbows, draw your shoulders through your legs. Tip your head down and lift your buttocks high up into the air. Now press your inner thighs firmly into your upper arms and shoulders and press your hands strongly into the mat, in preparation for sitting your buttocks down.

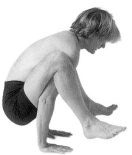

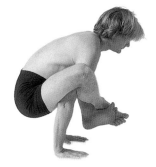

◀ 5 Still inhaling

(Vinyasa 7) Pressing through the palms of your hands, lift up strongly through your arms, engage your bandhas, and as you lift your feet cross your right foot over your left. (Advanced) Jump to this position from Downward-facing Dog. When you first learn this pose, remain balanced here for five full breaths.

▲ 4 Still inhaling

(Beginner) Open up your chest and press your shoulders back into your thighs with an equal and opposite pressure to the legs. Using the counterbalancing forces, lift your head and extend your chest to lower your buttocks, and "sit" on the backs of your arms. Balance on your hands as your feet float into the air.

▶ 6 Exhaling (x 5 breaths)

(Vinyasa 8) Slowly exhaling, bend your elbows and, without allowing your legs or feet to contact the floor, touch the mat with your chin. At first you may have to tuck your head in and rest the top of your head on the mat. Try to keep your elbows directly over the heels of your hands and extend your buttocks back as you extend your chin forward. Now look to your nasagrai (nose) dristi and breathe deeply for five full breaths.

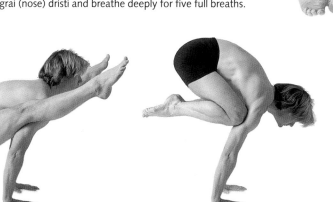

▲ 7– 8 Inhaling–Exhaling–Inhaling

(Vinyasa 9) Inhaling, lift your chin, uncross your feet, straighten your arms and legs into *Tittibhasana*, and look up. Exhale as you pivot at the knees to take your lower legs back, balancing on the back of your upper arms in *Bakasana*. (Vinyasa 10) With the strength of your inhalation and uddiyana bandha, lift your knees off your arms (see p. 65). Prepare to shoot your legs back and your chest forward to land in *Chatvari* (see p. 24).

▼ 9 Vinyasa up

(Vinyasas 11–15) Flow through this sequence of moves to finish in *Samasthitih* (see p. 67).

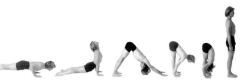

Sequence 2:
Tortoise and Sleeping Tortoise
Kurmasana and Supta Kurmasana

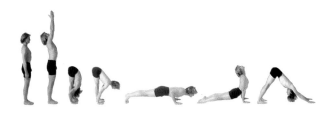

Kurma means "tortoise" and *supta* is "sleeping". This posture resembles the shape of a tortoise, first with its head and legs extended out from its shell and then, second, with its head and legs retracted to protect itself while asleep. The very nature of a tortoise is slow – an indication that this posture is not to be rushed. Take the time you need to learn the dynamics of these two complex postures, since the understanding that comes from them is vital for the completion of the second half of Yoga Chikitsa (body cleansing and purification). In addition, this asana is the "gateway" pose to Nadi Shodhana, or purification of the nervous system (*see p. 15*).

This asana begins to work on the subtle body by stimulating the *kanda* (nerve plexus). The kanda is located in the lower abdomen, where the body's thousands of nadis (energy channels/nerves) originate. The Tortoise pose has a purifying effect on the heart and lungs. The opening of your hip joints coming from work in earlier postures is necessary here, allowing you to place your legs over the back of your shoulders and neck.

By placing the weight of your legs on the back of your neck you develop extra strength through your entire spine – and this strength is important for the following asanas. Your chest is broadened, too, breathing difficulties are corrected, and when you are able to balance the strength and length of your inhalations and exhalations, your respiratory system can develop to its full potential.

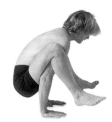

▲ **1 Vinyasa down**
(Vinyasas 1–6) Flow through this sequence of moves to Downward-facing Dog (*see p. 64*).

▲ **2 Inhaling**
From Downward-facing Dog, jump up into the air to the point of balance and bring your legs around the outside of your arms, landing on the backs of your arms, as shown on page 99, step 4.

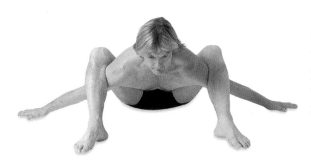

◀ 3 Still inhaling

Bending your elbows, lower your self down on to the mat and stretch your arms out to the sides from under your legs. Continue until the backs of your knees are well over your shoulders. At this point, do not put any pressure on the backs of your elbows.

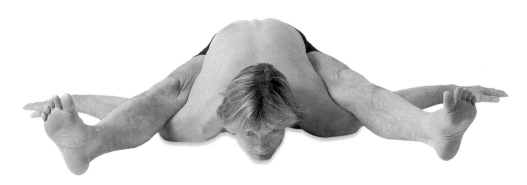

▲ 4 Inhaling (x 5 breaths)

(Vinyasa 7) Roll your pubic bone toward the mat and, lengthening from your pubic bone to your sternum, bring your chest to the mat. Widen out through your collar bones and out through your arms to your fingertips, and extend your chin forward. Now straighten your legs, pulling up on your kneecaps and thighs. Look to your broomadhya (third eye) dristi and breathe deeply for five full breaths.

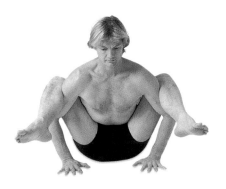

◀ 5 Inhaling

At this point, you learn the transition into *Supta Kurmasana* by your teacher adjusting the detail of your pose. It is possible, however, to release yourself from *Kurmasana* and to put your legs (left one first), one at a time, behind your head. Or you can bend your knees, drawing your heels in to create a space to place your hands on the mat, a shoulder-distance apart. Press firmly through your palms and lift your legs off the mat to roll back on to your buttocks.

(For the rest of the sequence turn to next page.)

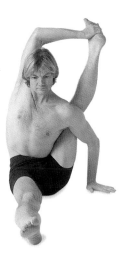

◀ **6 Exhaling–Inhaling**

Exhaling, release your right leg and take hold of your left foot with your right hand. Inhaling, press firmly through your left hand, pushing your left shoulder back into your left thigh. Keeping your spine straight and your pelvis square, straighten your left leg. Feel the stretch through the entire length of your leg.

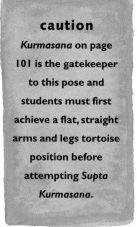

caution

Kurmasana on page 101 is the gatekeeper to this pose and students must first achieve a flat, straight arms and legs tortoise position before attempting *Supta Kurmasana.*

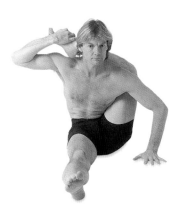

◀ **7 Exhaling**

Bend your left leg and, rotating your hip joint, turn your left knee outward. As you fold your leg behind your head, draw the left side of your torso past your left thigh. To keep your left leg located behind your head, sit tall through your spine, press back with your left shoulder, and lift your head. Now release your right hand.

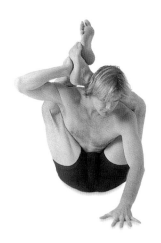

◀ **8 Inhaling–Exhaling**

(Vinyasa 8) Inhaling, maintain your balance by placing your left hand forward. Then hook your right leg over the back of your right arm and take hold of your ankle with your right hand. Exhaling, lift your right calf muscle with your right thumb and slip your left foot under the ankle of your right foot. Again, draw the side of your torso past your right thigh. Now flex both feet to lock your legs behind your head. Lift your head and broaden your chest.

▶ 9 Exhaling (x 5 breaths)

(Vinyasa 9) Release your right hand and place it on the mat and slowly lower yourself down to rest on your forehead. Extend your arms out to the sides and, rotating in your shoulder joints, fold your arms up behind your back. Hold your left wrist with your right hand. Keep your bandhas fully engaged, look to broomadhya (third eye) dristi, and breathe deeply for five full breaths.

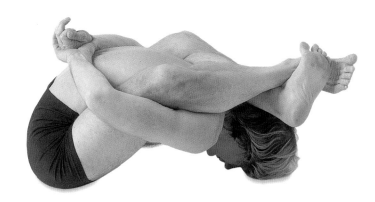

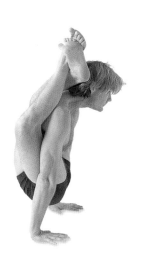

◀ 10–11 Exhaling (x 5 breaths)

Exhaling, release your binding and place your hands on the mat just under your shoulders. Press firmly through the palms of your hands and begin to lift your head off the floor. (Vinyasa 10) Inhaling, using the strength of your arms and bandhas, lift your body off the mat. To keep your legs located behind your head, continue to look to broomadhya dristi as you strongly press your head backward. Breathe deeply for five full breaths.

▶ 12–13 Inhaling–Exhaling–Inhaling

Inhaling, unlock your feet and straighten your arms and legs into Firefly (*Tittibhasana*), and look up. Exhaling, pivot at your knees and take your lower legs back, balancing on the back of your upper arms, into Crane (*Bakasana*). (Vinyasa 11) With the strength of your inhalation and uddiyana bandha, lift your knees off your arms (*see p. 65*). Prepare to shoot your legs back and your chest forward to land in *Chatvari* (*see p. 24*).

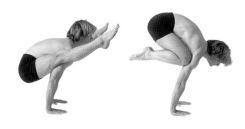

▶ 14 Vinyasa up

(Vinyasas 12–16) Flow through this sequence of moves to finish in *Samasthitih* (*see p. 67*).

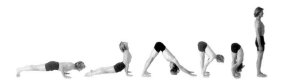

Sequence 2:

Fetus in the Womb and Rooster
Garbha Pindasana and Kukkutasana

Garbha means "womb", *pinda* is "fetus", and *kukku* translates as "rooster". These two postures come at the climax of the Yoga Chikitsa series, at which stage your body is generating optimum working heat. Breath bandhas and vinyasas have created such an internal fire that you sweat from every pore, and it is this that provides the lubrication you need. This sequence provides many benefits, the main one being the pressure it places on your spleen and liver. This massages toxins out of these organs, producing a cleansing effect. The rocking and rolling motion is also excellent for your entire spine, releasing any tension that may have developed in the Tortoise sequence. The rocking and rolling and the lifting on to your hands further develops inner body control.

> **tip**
> If you do not produce enough lubricating sweat to allow your arms to slip through your legs, ask an assistant to lightly spray your body with water from a plant mister.

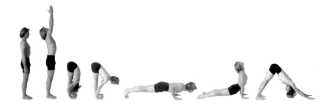

◄ **1 Vinyasa down**
(Vinyasas 1–6) Flow through this sequence of moves to Downward-facing Dog (see p. 64).

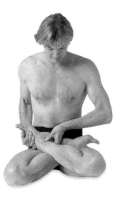

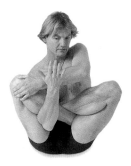

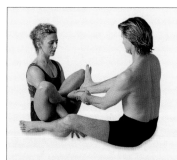

▲ **2 Inhaling**
From Downward-facing Dog, jump through your arms to *Dandasana* and fold your legs into *Padmasana* (Lotus), right leg first. Bear in mind that it is the space between your Achilles and thighs that you will be sliding your arms through.

▲ **3 Still inhaling**
Using your left hand as a support, hold your fingers straight like a knife and, aiming your forearm to the left, slide your right hand and forearm through your right lotus, just in front of your left ankle. Reversing lefts and rights, do the same with your other arm.

If you need help to achieve this position, using one foot as a stabilizer, your partner braces the other against the underside of your knee. This arrangement leaves both hands free to pull your arm through your leg. Your partner reverses legs positions to pull your other arm through.

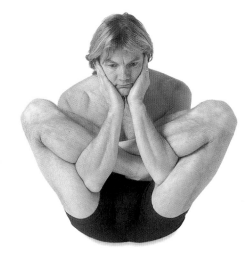

◀ 4 Inhaling (x 5 breaths)

(Vinyasa 7) Flex your left arm to bring your elbow through, and then draw your hands in to cup your face. Balancing entirely on the bones in your rump, lengthen from your pubic bone to sternum and open up your chest region. Look to nasagrai (nose) dristi and breathe deeply for five full breaths. If you manage to close off your ears with your fingers, the internal sound of your breath is similar to the sounds a fetus hears while in the womb.

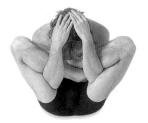

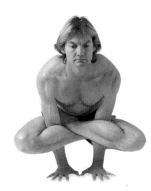

◀ 6 Inhaling–Exhaling

Twist your buttocks slightly to the right to help you rotate clockwise and roll up forward, along the line of your spine as you inhale. Exhaling, roll backward, again twisting your buttocks to the right. Repeat this a total of nine times to complete a full circle, finishing with your spine aligned with the middle line of the mat.

▲ 5 Exhaling

(Vinyasa 8) Tuck your head down into your hands and shorten the distance between your sternum and pubic bone as you curl up into a ball. Make sure you round your spine – any flat spot will impede the rolling action. Continue to exhale as you roll backward along the line of your spine.

◀ 7 Inhaling (x 5 breaths)

(Vinyasa 9) On the last roll up, use the force of the inhalation to initiate *Kukkutasana* – place your hands flat down and straighten your arms to lift your body off the floor. Open up your chest, lift your head, and look to nasagrai (nose) dristi. Breathe deeply for five full breaths.

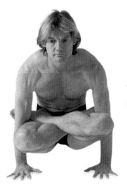

◀ 8 Inhaling

(Vinyasa 10) Slide your arms out, placing your hands to the sides of your lotus, press firmly through your palms, and lift your body off the mat. Engage your bandhas and swing your lotus through your arms. At the point of balance, release your lotus and prepare to shoot your legs back and your chest forward to land in *Chatvari* (see p. 24).

▼ 9 Vinyasa up

(Vinyasas 11–15) Flow through this sequence of moves to finish in *Samasthitih* (see p. 67).

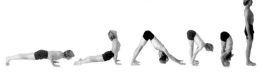

Sequence 2:
Bound Angle
Baddha Konasana

Baddha means "bound" and *kona* is "angle". This posture is sometimes called Cobbler's Seat. Yoga texts consider *Baddha Konasana* as the greatest of asanas, claiming it cures diseases related to the anus. To achieve the therapeutic benefits, mula bandha and uddiyana bandha must be engaged. On a more physical level, this posture opens your hips and it is the counterpose to *Bhujapidasana* and *Kurmasana (see pp. 98–9 and 100–103)*. Achieving the Bound Angle may come easily to those students who have spent many years sitting on the floor. However, those who habitually sit in chairs or have played very physical sports may experience some difficulty and perhaps discomfort or even pain while learning it. Because of this, you need to practise *Baddha Konasana* with sensitivity and understanding.

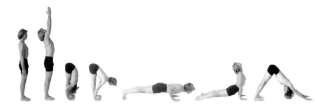

◀ **1 Vinyasa down**
(Vinyasas 1–6) Flow through this sequence of moves to Downward-facing Dog (*see p. 64*).

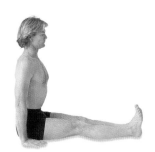

▲ **2 Inhaling**
From Downward-facing Dog, jump through your arms to *Dandasana*. Sit tall through your spine and fully engage mula and uddiyana bandhas, as described on page 71, step 6.

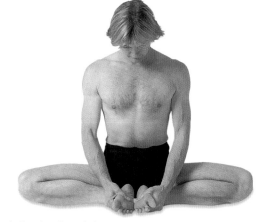

▲ **3 Inhaling (x 5 breaths)**
(Vinyasa 7) Bend your knees and draw your heels in to press against the perineum. Join your feet, turning your soles up (like opening up a book). Now, releasing your hip joints, press your knees to the mat. Continue activating your bandhas, lift your chest, and lengthen your spine. Look to nasagrai (nose) dristi and breathe deeply for five full breaths.

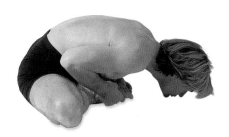

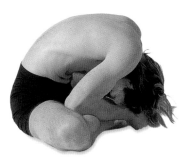

▲ 4 Exhaling (x 5 breaths)

(Vinyasa 8) Maintaining the extension in your spine, roll your pubic bone toward the floor and, folding forward from your hip joints, place your chin on the mat. Look to nasagrai (nose) dristi and breathe deeply for five full breaths. Relax your shoulders and, working with the directional energy of uddiyana bandha, continue to lengthen the space between your pubic bone and sternum with each inhalation. On each exhalation, reinforce the application of mula bandha.

▲ 5 Inhaling (x 5 breaths)

Inhaling, release the forward stretching and sit tall. Exhaling, contract inward from your abdomen, and curl your spine down so that you can place the top of your head on the soles of your feet. Continue looking to nasagrai (nose) dristi and breathe deeply for five full breaths. Stretch through the back of your neck in preparation for the next position.

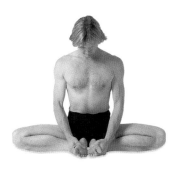

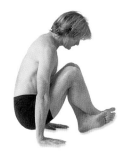

◀ 7 Exhaling–Inhaling

Exhaling, release your hands, cross your legs and place your hands a shoulder-distance apart on the mat, just forward of your hip joints. (Vinyasa 10) Inhaling, press firmly through the palms of your hands, lean forward, lift your body off the mat, and swing your legs through your arms, and prepare to land in *Chatvari* (see p. 24).

▲ 6 Inhaling

(Vinyasa 9) Sit tall again, returning to the position described in step 3.

▼ 8 Vinyasa up

(Vinyasas 11–15) Flow through this sequence of moves to finish in *Samasthitih* (see p. 67).

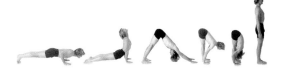

Sequence 2:
Seated Angle
Upavishta Konasana

Upavishta means "seated", and *kona* translates as "angle". This sequence of movements is the seated version of the standing, wide-angle postures of the *Prasarita Padottanasana* variations (*see pp. 50–9*). Here, with a change of foundation, the sciatic nerve is intensely stretched, strengthening it along with the other nerves that originate in the spine and travel through to the legs. Your spinal column, lower back, and waist are all strengthened as a result. The application of mula and uddiyana bandhas is very important, not only to retain and direct the internal energy but also to prevent any overstretching of the hamstrings and sciatic nerve. The second component of this asana is the elevation of the posture – a lift that requires a sense of balance that is a true test of the quality of bandha application.

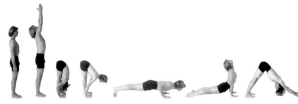

◀ **1 Vinyasa down**
(Vinyasas 1–6) Flow through this sequence of moves to Downward-facing Dog (*see p. 64*).

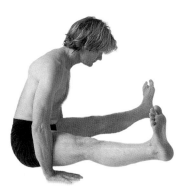

▲ **2 Inhaling**
From Downward-facing Dog, jump your legs through your arms without allowing your body or legs to touch the mat. Open your legs wide and slowly lower yourself down on to the mat.

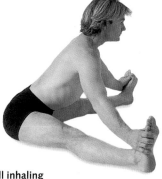

▲ **3 Still inhaling**
(Vinyasa 7) Straighten your legs and reach forward with your arms to take hold of the outside edges of your feet. Press your thumb on the point between the base of the big and second toe of each foot. Open up, lifting your chest away from your legs until your arms and back are straight. Lengthen the region between your pubic bone and sternum and look up to your broomadhya (third eye) dristi.

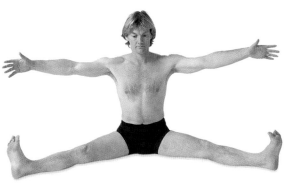

▲ 4 Exhaling (x 5 breaths)

(Vinyasa 8) Draw your lower abdomen in to maintain the length in your lower back, roll your pubic bone toward the floor, and fold down, placing your chin on the mat. Pull up on your kneecaps and thighs, roll your inner thigh muscles up toward the sky, and extend the stretch from your groin to your ankles. Draw your torso forward, extending out through your chin. Look to broomadhya (third eye) dristi and breathe deeply for five full breaths.

▲ 5 Inhaling

(Beginner/intermediate) Release your hands, lift your head and torso, and raise your arms to shoulder height. (Eventually you will find it possible to lift your legs to the balance point shown in step 6.)

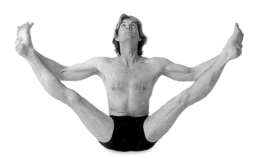

▲ 6 inhaling (x 5 breaths)

(Vinyasa 9) Keeping your legs straight, lift them off the floor and up to your waiting hands (advanced). Catch the outside edge of your feet. Draw in your lower abdomen and roll your pubic bone forward to bring your pelvis to the critical balance point. Lift your chest, look to urdhva (up to the sky) dristi, and breathe deeply for five full breaths.

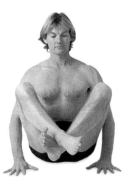

◀ 7 Exhaling–Inhaling

Exhaling, release your hands, cross your legs without allowing your feet to touch the floor, and place your hands, a shoulder-distance apart, on the mat just forward of your hip joints. (Vinyasa 10) Inhaling, press firmly through the palms of your hands, lean forward, lift your body off the mat, and swing your legs through your arms and then back to *Chatvari (see p. 24).*

▶ 8 Vinyasa up

(Vinyasas 11–15) Flow through this sequence of moves to finish in *Samasthitih (see p. 67).*

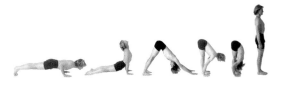

Sequence 2:

Sleeping Angle
Supta Konasana

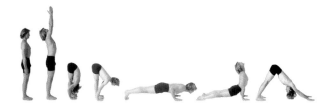

Supta means "sleeping" and *kona* translates as "angle". This asana is the first of the inverted asanas and it is the initial preparation for *Salamba Sarvangasana* (*see pp.128–9*), and the prerequisite for *Chakrasana* (*see pp. 114–15*). The entry to this asana is from a prone *Samasthitih* (*see p. 24*). There is also an extra exhalation in this position to engage the bandhas. The use of bandha control is crucial, first, to protect your lower back and, second, to initiate the internal energy you need to lift your legs off the floor. Neck muscles are strengthened as you push with the back of your head to start the rolling-up momentum, and the muscles along the entire length of your spine are massaged.

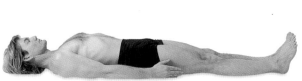

◀ **1 Vinyasa down**
(Vinyasas 1–6) Flow through this sequence of moves to Downward-facing Dog (*see p. 64*).

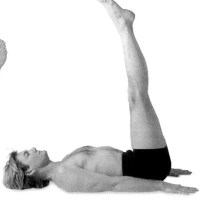

▲ **2 Inhaling–Exhaling**
(Vinyasa 7) From Downward-facing Dog, inhaling, jump through your arms to *Dandasana* and look to your toes dristi. Exhaling, hold the sides of your thighs with your hands and, curving your spine, roll down, one vertebra at a time, until your back is completely flat on the mat. Before you lower your head, check the alignment of your spine and make any corrections necessary to centre your body on your mid line. Pull up on your kneecaps and thighs, engage your bandha control, and straighten your arms. This is not a resting or relaxing position, however: in essence it is *Samasthitih*, except that you are lying down.

▲ **3 Inhaling**
Roll your arms inward, toward your body, and place your hands flat on the mat beside your thighs. Now, using the internal energy harnessed by the application of the bandhas, lift your straight legs off the mat and up into the air. Directing the internal lift up through your legs, and with a push from your arms, lift your buttocks and back off the mat as well.

▶ **4 Exhaling (x 5 breaths)**

(Vinyasa 8) Exhaling, roll up on to your shoulders, bring your legs over your head to the floor, open them out, and hold your big toes with the first two fingers of each of your hands. Straighten your legs and back to lengthen the space between your pubic bone and sternum. Look to nasagrai (nose) dristi and breathe deeply for five full breaths. At the end of the last exhalation, flex further into the back of the neck – as if you were drawing a bow string back.

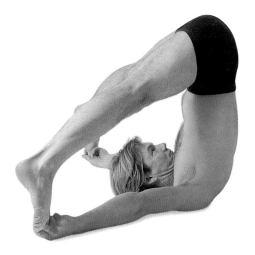

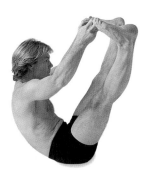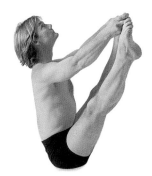

▲ **5–6 Inhaling**

Engage your bandhas, push with the back of your head, and begin to roll up along the length of your spine. Keep your chin tucked in toward your sternum as you roll and, just as you reach the balance point, open up and lift your head and chest. Look up to broomadhya (third eye) dristi. Maintain this balance for the split second between the end of this inhalation and the beginning of the next exhalation.

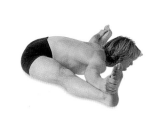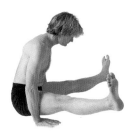

▲ **7–8 Exhaling–Inhaling–Exhaling**

(Vinyasa 9) Exhaling, slowly lower down into step 4 of Seated Angle on page 109. (Vinyasa 10) Inhaling, lift your head up and, exhaling, place your hands down on the mat beside your thighs. Press firmly through the palms of your hands. (Vinyasa 11) Inhaling, lift your entire body off the mat and cross your legs. Exhaling, swing your legs back through your arms to land in *Chatvari* (see p. 24).

▶ **9 Vinyasa up**

(Vinyasas 12–16) Flow through this sequence of moves to finish in *Samasthitih* (see p. 67).

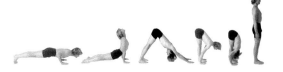

Sequence 2:

Lying Down Leg Raises
Supta Padangusthasana

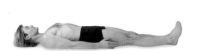 *Supta* means "sleeping", *pada* is "foot", and *angustha* translates as "big toe". This asana is the prone version of the standing leg raises (*see pp. 60–1*) and, once again, entry into it is from the prone version of *Samasthitih* (*see pp. 38 and 110*). This is a very difficult posture, since you are, in effect, standing while lying down. The difficulty here does not lie in balance; rather, it is finding the connection to your foundation. The ground has been taken away from under your "standing" foot and so the use of bandha control is important in rooting you down into an internal foundation. The "standing" leg, therefore, has to be worked strongly – just as if you were standing. The use of bandha control will ground the posture and protect your lower back.

> **tip**
> To maintain the necessary central axis through this posture, it is important to check the alignment of your spine and to engage your bandhas while lying down.

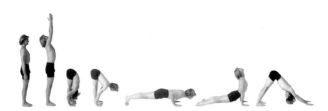

◀ **1 Vinyasa down**
(Vinyasas 1–6) Flow through this sequence of moves to Downward-facing Dog (*see p. 64*).

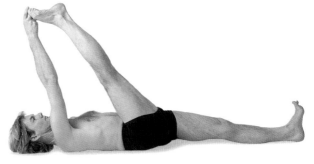

▲ **2 Inhaling–Exhaling**
(Vinyasa 7) From Downward-facing Dog, inhaling, jump through your arms to *Dandasana*. Exhaling, check the line of your spine as you lie down, as described on page 110, step 2.

▲ **3 Inhaling**
(Vinyasa 8) Place your left hand on your left thigh – this is your "standing" leg. Engage your bandhas both to protect your lower back and to hold your pelvis square. Now, drawing on your internal energy source, raise your right leg straight up. Hold the big toe of your right leg with the first two fingers of your right hand and look up to your padhayoragrai (foot) dristi.

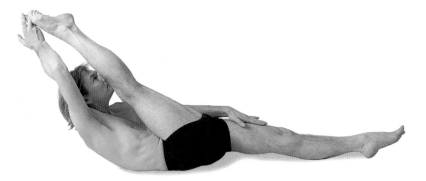

▲ 4 Exhaling (x 5 breaths)

(Vinyasa 9) Exhaling, push strongly down through your left leg, as if standing on it, and raise your back completely off the mat. Lift with the strength of the upper abdominals, combined with bandhas, and touch your chin to your shin. Using the opposing energies between your right arm and right leg to hold your back off the mat, look to padhayoragrai dristi and breathe deeply for five full breaths.

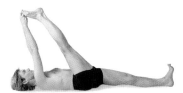

◀ 5 Inhaling

(Vinyasa 10) Keep both of your legs activated and lower your back and head down to the mat – resuming the same position described in step 3.

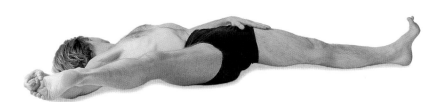

▲ 6 Exhaling (x 5 breaths)

(Vinyasa 11) Continuing the engagement of mula and uddiyana bandhas, press your left hand firmly on your left thigh to keep your pelvis square and level. Exhaling, release your right hip joint and rotate your right leg out to the right side and bring it down to the mat. Roll your inner thigh down and rest your heel on the mat. Then draw your abdomen in, strengthen both legs, and lengthen through your spine. Rotate your head to look over your left shoulder to parsva dristi, and breathe deeply for five full breaths.

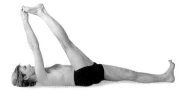

◀ 7 Inhaling

(Vinyasa 12) Press firmly through your left hand and raise your right leg back up to the vertical plane, as described in step 3.

(For the rest of the sequence turn to next page.)

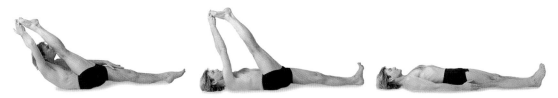

▲ **8–9–10 Exhaling–Inhaling–Exhaling**

(Vinyasa 13) Exhaling, lift your back off the mat and touch your chin to your shin, as in step 4, page 113. (Vinyasa 14) Inhaling, lower your back and head back down to the mat, as in step 3, page 112. (Vinyasa 15) Exhaling, lower your right leg back down to the mat and return to the neutral lying down position of step 2. From this point (step 2), repeat the following steps for the left leg (vinyasas 16–23), reversing the directions for rights and lefts.

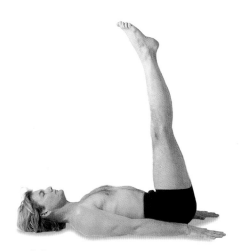

▲ **11 Inhaling**

After completing the left side, initiate *Chakrasana*, or the Backward Roll. Place your hands flat on the mat beside your thighs and, using the internal energy harnessed by the bandhas, lift your straight legs off the mat and into the air. Directing the internal lift up through your legs toward the sky, and with a push from your arms on the mat, lift your buttocks and back off the floor. This initial lifting action is important to develop, since it is the same action required to lift up into the Shoulder Stand (*see pp. 128–31*).

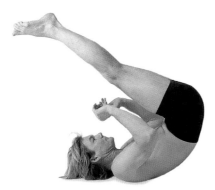

◀ 12 Still inhaling

(*Chakrasana*) Continue lifting your back off the mat, bringing your legs over your head at about a 45° angle. Raise your arms from their flat position on the mat to a position over your head. Breath and movement synchronicity, the essence of vinyasa, is vital here (*see pp. 18–23*) to convert the internal lifting action and rolling momentum into a graceful backward roll.

▶ 13 Still inhaling

(*Chakrasana*) Flowing with the rolling momentum of step 12, place your hands over on to the mat either side of your head with your fingers pointing toward your shoulders. At the exact time that you roll on to the point of your shoulders, press firmly through your palms. Keeping your legs energized and, synchronous with the push through your palms, shoot your legs backward. The rolling momentum combined with the lift through your legs and the push from your hands will provide enough space to clear your head. At this point, do not abort the full *Chakrasana* by dipping one shoulder or tipping your head to one side – this could hurt your neck. You must develop the inner lift and the synchronicity of the push through your hands with the flowing inhalation.

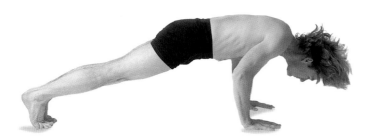

▲ 14 Exhaling

(*Chakrasana*) At exactly the same time as you shoot your legs backward and push with your hands, described in step 13, swing your head through the space between your arms, landing on the balls of your feet. Bend your elbows close into the sides of your torso and lower yourself down into *Chatvari* – vinyasa 4 of *Surya Namaskara* A (*see pp. 24–5*). Look to nasagrai (nose) dristi.

▼ 15 Vinyasa up

(Vinyasas 24–28) After completing the Backward Roll shown in detail above, flow through this sequence of moves to finish in *Samasthitih* (*see p. 67*).

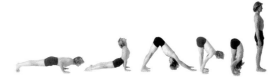

Sequence 2:
Both Big Toes
Ubhaya Padangusthasana

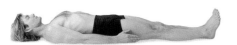

Ubhaya means "both", *pada* is "foot", and *angustha* means "big toe". This asana is the same as *Supta Konasana*, or Sleeping Angle (*see pp. 110–11*), except that the angle has been closed, bringing both legs together. This asana is particularly beneficial in purifying and strengthening the waist, stomach, anus, and genitals. The push from the back of the head and the rolling action of the entry into this asana strengthen and prepare your spine for the closing posture of the Yoga Chikitsa series, The Bridge (*see pp. 120–1*), and the finishing postures (*see pp. 128–33*). The grace that can be achieved in the straight-leg entry into this asana demonstrates the internal energy that is harnessed by the application of mula and uddiyana bandhas.

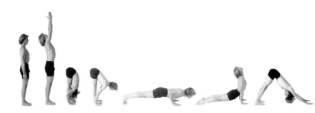

◀ **1 Vinyasa down**
(Vinyasas 1–6) Flow through this sequence of moves to Downward-facing Dog (*see p. 64*).

▲ **2 Inhaling–Exhaling**
(Vinyasa 7) From Downward-facing Dog, inhaling, jump through your arms to *Dandasana* and then, exhaling, check the line of your spine as you lie down, as described on page 110, step 2.

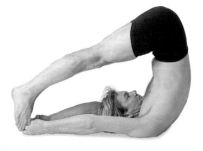

▲ **3 Inhaling**
(Vinyasa 8) Place your hands on the mat beside your thighs. Using the internal energy of the bandhas, lift your straight legs off the mat. With a push from your arms, lift your buttocks and back and roll up on to your shoulders. Bring your legs over your head to the mat and hold your big toes with the first two fingers of each hand. Straighten and lengthen your legs and back, and look to nasagrai (nose) dristi.

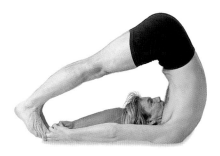

◄ 4 Exhaling

As if drawing back a bow string, flex further into the back of your neck. Make sure you use the full length of your exhalation and, at the end of the exhalation, draw your lower abdomen in and engage your mula bandha and uddiyana bandha. Continue looking to nasagrai dristi to bring your focus deeper into your inner body control.

▶ 5 Inhaling

(Vinyasa 9) Push strongly with the back of your head and begin to roll up along the length of your spine. Keep your chin tucked in toward your sternum and allow your spine to form a curve. The technique here is to hold your toes very lightly to bridge the opposing forces between the strength of your legs and arms. Now roll, leading from your navel, not your legs.

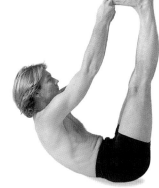

▶ 6 Exhaling (x 5 breaths)

If not controlled, this flowing, rolling momentum will take you past the point of balance. The technique for preventing this and stopping at the balance point is to exhale fully and, at precisely the same time, open up your chest and lift your head. Once you have established balance, look up to broomadhya (third eye) dristi. Maintaining your balance, breathe deeply for five full breaths.

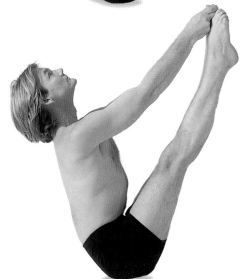

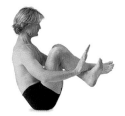 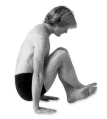

▲ 7–8 Exhaling–Inhaling

Release your toes, cross your legs without touching the mat, and draw them into your chest as you finish your exhalation. At the same time, with your hands poised, rock forward into your hands. (Vinyasa 10) Inhaling, keep your legs tucked in and off the mat and lift your body up. Then swing your legs back through your arms to land in Chatvari (see p. 24).

▼ 9 Vinyasa up

(Vinyasas 11–15) Flow through this sequence of moves to finish in Samasthitih (see p. 67).

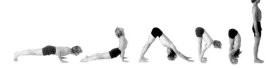

Sequence 2:

Balancing Forward Bend
Urdhva Mukha Paschimattanasana

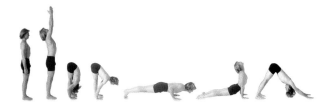

Urdhva means "upward", *mukha* is "face", *paschima* is "west", and *uttana* translates as "intense". The challenge of this sequence is to develop the ability to balance with grace and poise while adopting an extreme pose. This sequence follows on from the previous one and shares its therapeutic benefits. To practise it correctly, and achieve inner peace, an appreciation of mula and uddiyana bandhas needs to be established. As we come to the end of Yoga Chikitsa, we repeat the dynamic counterpose combination of an intense forward bend followed by an intense back bend. The balancing postures demonstrate the advanced level of yoga asana, which can be achieved when asanas are grouped in a specific order. If followed strictly, this order will improve and cleanse the joint, muscle, nerve, and organ functions.

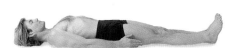

◀ **1 Vinyasa down**
(Vinyasas 1–6) Flow through this sequence of moves to Downward-facing Dog (*see p. 64*).

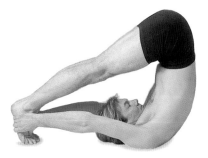

▲ **2 Inhaling–Exhaling**
(Vinyasa 7) From Downward-facing Dog, inhaling, jump through your arms to *Dandasana* and, exhaling, check the line of your spine as you lie down, as described on page 110, step 2.

▲ **3 Inhaling–Exhaling**
(Vinyasa 8) Place your hands on the mat beside your thighs and, using the internal energy of the bandhas, lift your straight legs up. With a push from your arms, lift your buttocks and back and roll on to your shoulders. Bring your legs over your head to the mat, and grip the sides of your feet. Straighten your legs and back. Look to nasagrai dristi. Now, exhaling, flex further into the back of your neck. Engage your bandhas and prepare to roll up on the next inhalation.

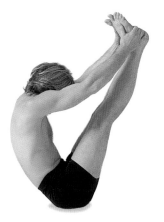

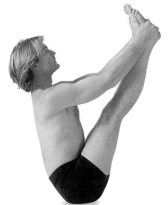

▲ 4 Inhaling

(Vinyasa 9) Push strongly with the back of your head and begin to roll up along the length of your spine. Keep your chin tucked in toward your sternum and allow your spine to form a curve. Hold your feet very lightly to bridge the opposing forces between the strength of your legs and arms. Now start to roll – leading from your navel, not your legs.

◀ 5 Still inhaling

(Vinyasa 9) Continue to roll up with straight legs and balance on the sit bones. To hold this point of balance, keep your legs straight and point your toes upward. Now straighten your arms, open up your chest, and lift your head. Draw your abdomen in and look to your padhayoragrai (toes) dristi.

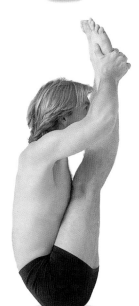

◀ 6 Exhaling (x 5 breaths)

(Vinyasa 10) Release your knees and slightly bend them. Roll your pubic bone through toward the back of your thighs to gain lift out of your lower back, extend your torso up along your vertical legs, and bring your chin into your shins. Pull up on your kneecaps and thighs to straighten your legs, look to padhayoragrai dristi, and focus inwardly on your mula and uddiyana bandhas. Maintain this balance and breathe deeply for five full breaths.

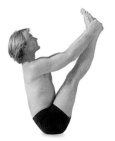
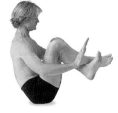

▲ 7–8–9 Inhaling–Exhaling–Inhaling

Inhaling, open up to the position in step 5. Exhaling, release your feet and cross your legs without touching the mat, drawing them into your chest as you finish the exhalation. At the same time, with hands poised in the air, rock forward into your hands. (Vinyasa 11) Inhaling, keeping your legs tucked in and off the mat, lift your body up and then swing your legs back through your arms to land in *Chatvari* (see p. 24).

▼ 10 Vinyasa up

(Vinyasas 12–16) Flow through this sequence of moves to finish in *Samasthitih* (see p. 67).

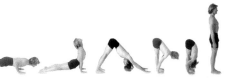

Sequence 2:
The Bridge
Setu Bandhasana

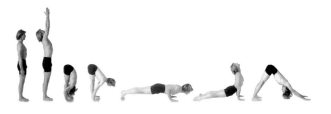

Setu means "bridge" and *bandha* translates as "lock", "seal", or "completion". This last asana of Yoga Chikitsa (*see p. 15*) is a counterpose to the previous group, which stretched aspects of the neck and spine. *Setu Bandhasana* is a combination of balance and strength, and it acts as the bridge between the forward bending asana you have just completed and the back bends that follow. As the neck is extended backwards, the top of your head and feet become the foundations for your body. Your neck muscles become stronger and more elastic as a result, and your legs and back have to work strongly to support your frame.

> **tip**
> The essential elements of back bending are introduced here in preparation for the more testing sequences to follow.

◀ **1 Vinyasa down**
(Vinyasas 1–6) Flow through this sequence of moves to Downward-facing Dog (*see p. 64*).

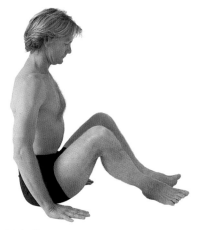

▲ **2 Inhaling**
(Vinyasa 7) From Downward-facing Dog, jump through your arms to *Dandasana*. Then, bending your knees, draw your feet in until they are about 45cm (18in) from your pubic bone. Place your heels together, turn your toes outward, and place your feet on the mat, Charlie Chaplin fashion. Look to your feet.

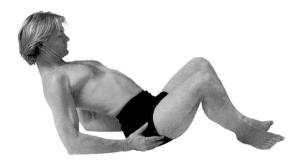

▲ **3 Exhaling**
(Vinyasa 8) Hold the sides of your buttocks with your hands and lie back, taking the weight on to your elbows. Roll your pubic bone down toward the floor, lengthen through your abdomen, and lift your chest. Continue to look to your feet to ensure that the line from your heels to your chin is straight as it can be as you lie back.

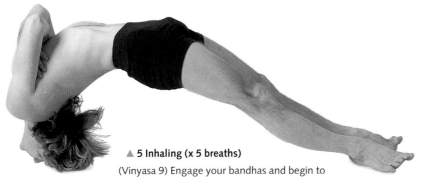

◀ 4 Still exhaling
(Vinyasa 8) Push on your elbows and continuing to arch your spine. Take your head back, placing the top of your head on the mat. Now press down a little with your head and release your hands from the sides of your buttocks. Next, cross your arms and place your hands under your armpits. Equalize the foundation pressure between your feet, buttocks, and head. Look to your nasagrai (nose) dristi.

▲ 5 Inhaling (x 5 breaths)
(Vinyasa 9) Engage your bandhas and begin to press more strongly through your feet and head to release your buttock foundation. The foundation must be firm and equal in both feet and head before lifting your buttocks off the mat. Now lift strongly through your legs and upper spine. Continue looking to your nasagrai dristi to maintain a straight central axis. Once you are stable and your buttocks are off the mat, pull up on your kneecaps and thighs to fully straighten your legs. Equalize the push with your head, and roll from the top of your head to your forehead. Maintain your balance and breathe deeply for five full breaths.

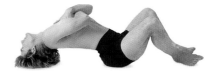

▲ 6 Exhaling
(Vinyasa 10) Intensify the focus on your head foundation and slowly begin to bend your knees. Maintain an equal pressure between your head and feet as you roll back down along the centre line of your crown to the same position as in step 4.

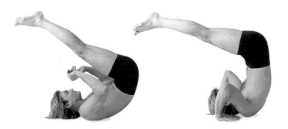

▲ 7–8 Inhaling
Release your crossed arms and place your hands back at the sides of you buttocks so that you can lift and release your head and neck. Using the internal energy harnessed by the bandhas; lift your legs off the mat and into the air. Rolling into *Chakrasana*, or Backward Roll (*see pp.114–15*), shoot your legs backward and land in *Chatvari* (*see p. 24*).

▼ 9 Vinyasa up
(Vinyasas 11–15) After completing the Backward Roll shown above, flow through this sequence of moves to finish in *Samasthitih* (*see p. 67*).

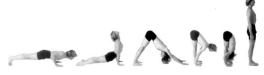

Sequence 2:
Back Bending
Urdhva Dhanurasana

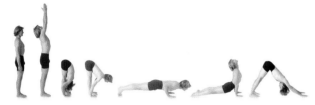

Urdhva means "upward" and *dhanura* is "bow". The work of Yoga Chikitsa has focused mainly on internal cleansing and the correction of muscular/skeletal imbalances through forward-bending postures. Although many people have naturally flexible spines, they don't necessarily have the internal bandha control and leg strength required for back bends. However, if you have reached the end of the primary series, you should now be ready to begin. Here again you need your foot foundations, but your hands and legs will be working in an entirely new way. The emphasis is now on stretching and lengthening your quadriceps, opening your groin, abdomen, and chest and, hence, stretching the front, rather than the back, of the body.

◀ 1 Vinyasa down
(Vinyasas 1–6) Flow through this sequence of moves to Downward-facing Dog (*see p. 64*).

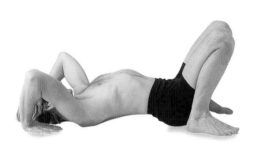

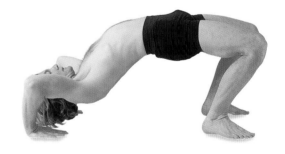

▲ 2 Exhaling
(Vinyasa 7) From Downward-facing Dog, jump through your arms to *Dandasana*. (Vinyasa 8) Exhaling, check the line of your spine as you lie down, straight as if in *Samasthitih*. Engage your bandhas and prepare your foundation for the upward bow by drawing your feet in toward your buttocks. Place them on the outsides of your hips and parallel. Place your hands on the mat either side of your head, a shoulder-distance apart, fingers spread and pointing backward.

▲ 3 Inhaling
(Vinyasa 9) Relax your buttocks, tuck your chin in toward your sternum, and, pressing with equal strength between your hands and feet foundations, lift your head, buttocks, and shoulders off the mat. To avoid jamming your lower back, and to balance your body's weight evenly between your hands/feet foundations, it is important to lift your shoulders off the mat at exactly the same time as your buttocks.

▶ **4 Inhaling (x 5 breaths)**

(Vinyasa 9) Continue to keep your buttocks relaxed as you lift into the upward bow. Use the strength in your arms and legs only – do not grip with your buttocks, as this will limit the opening in your groin. With equal force, push through the palms of your hands and the soles of your feet, open your chest, and relax the back of your neck. Look to your nasagrai (nose) dristi and breathe deeply for five full breaths.

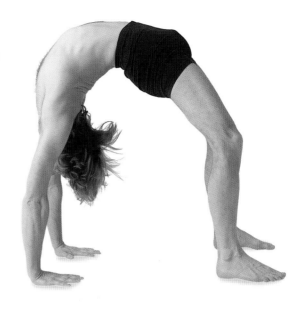

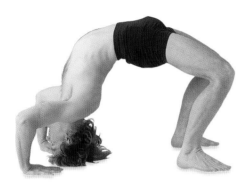

▲ **5 Exhaling–Inhaling**

Exhaling, slowly lower yourself down on to the top of your head. Take some of your body weight on to your new head foundation and remain like this for three full breaths. If your back is supple, transfer more weight on to your hands and head and walk your feet a little closer to your hand foundation.

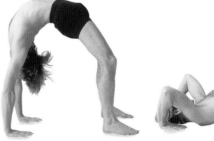

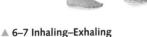

▲ **6–7 Inhaling–Exhaling**

Again, pressing with equal pressure between your hands and feet foundations, relax your neck and buttocks and lift back up into the upward bow, and breathe deeply for another five full breaths. (Vinyasa 10) Exhaling, after three repetitions, lie down, release your hands and feet foundations, and prepare to perform *Chakrasana*, or Backward Roll (*see pp. 114–15*).

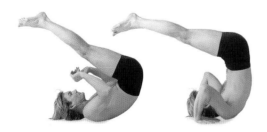

▲ **8–9 Inhaling**

Place your hands on the mat beside your buttocks, engage your bandhas, and, using the internal energy harnessed through bandha control, lift your legs off the mat and into the air. Rolling backward into *Chakrasana*, shoot your legs backward and land in *Chatvari* (*see p. 24*)

▼ **10 Vinyasa up**

(Vinyasas 11–15) After completing the Backward Roll, flow through this sequence of moves to finish in *Samasthitih* (*see p. 67*).

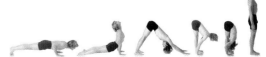

Sequence 2:
Advanced Back Bending
Urdhva Dhanurasana

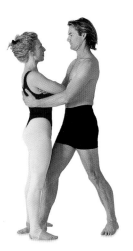

In the first back-bending sequence you established the new hands and feet foundations (*see pp. 122–3*) and began to develop the power and strength in your legs and arms needed to support your back in this position. The next step is to drop backward from standing into *Urdhva Dhanurasana*. Traditionally, Shri K Pattabhi Jois, at his yoga Shala (centre) in Mysore, India, introduces this sequence to students. It is crucial, therefore, to learn this sequence only from a qualified teacher. Allowing somebody to adjust you in a back drop requires trust. If this is not present you will tense your back and, so, defeat the point of the routine.

> **tip**
> This sequence will further develop leg strength and foundation. Once these are established, you can practise the back bend unassisted.

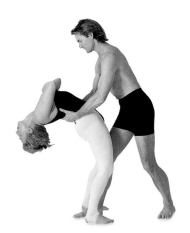

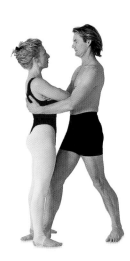

▲ **1– 2– 3 Inhaling–Exhaling– Inhaling**

From *Samasthitih*, inhaling, jump your feet a shoulder-distance apart and parallel. Stand tall with your tailbone tucked slightly in. Engage your bandhas and lengthen through the spine. Cross your arms, placing your hands under your armpits. Tuck your chin down and gaze to nasagrai dristi. As your teacher supports your back, exhaling, initiate the back bend from the feet foundation. Flex forward in your ankles, taking your shins over your toes. Leading with your tail and pubic bones, bring your pelvis forward of your foot foundation. Don't grip your buttocks. As you arch your back, keep looking to your nose dristi. Release your back into your teacher's hands and take your head back as you arch fully, opening the front side of your body. Inhaling, initiate your return to standing from your feet foundation. As if stretching the mat between your feet, stand strongly through the outsides of your thighs. Slowly straighten through your spine, allowing your head to return to the central axis last of all. Flowing with your breath, exhaling, repeat the above steps two more times.

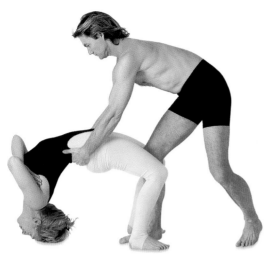

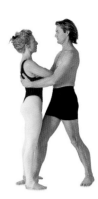

▶ 5 Inhaling

Your teacher will initiate the lift necessary to return you back to the standing position. As soon as you feel this, begin to lead forward with your pelvis and stand down into your legs.

▲ 4 Exhaling (x 5 breaths)

After the third repeat, the teacher takes you over, backward, to rest you on your forehead. Again, initiate the back bend as in steps 1 and 2, maintaining power in your legs. Once on your forehead, don't relax your legs, keep them working strongly. Look to nasagrai dristi and breathe deeply for five full breaths.

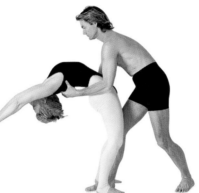

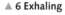

▲ 6 Exhaling

Prepare to drop on to your hands. Flexing forward in your ankles, bring your shins, knees, and pelvis forward of your toes. Lengthen out of your pelvis and begin to arch. Take your head back as you release into your teacher's hands and, just as you see the mat in your peripheral vision, release your hands from your armpits and stretch your arms out straight.

▲ 7 Still exhaling

Continue to arch backward until your hands reach the mat. Try to land on your fingers, and then your palms. Allow your elbows to act only as shock absorbers – don't let them bend too much as this will unbalance your body weight; gravity will then take over and your shoulders will become overloaded. Now repeat steps 5, 6, and 7 three times.

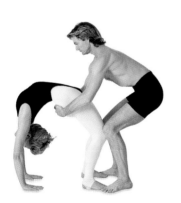

▲ 8 Inhaling (x 5 breaths)

Walk your hands a little closer to your feet. Don't lift your feet or turn your heels inward as this will inhibit the strength you can bring to bear through your legs. The teacher assists as you work into a deep bend. Breathe deeply for five breaths. Your teacher then initiates the return to standing.

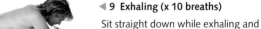

◀ 9 Exhaling (x 10 breaths)

Sit straight down while exhaling and immediately fold into a seated forward bend. The addition of your teacher's body weight will intensify the important counterstretching element of the movement. Exhaling, jump back to *Chatvari* (see p. 24) and then vinyasa up to *Samasthitih* (see p. 67).

Sequence 3:

The Finishing Sequence

This group of asanas is called the "finishing sequence" for the simple reason that all practitioners should conclude their asana practice with the following postures, and these should be carried out in the precise order they are presented in this part of the book. Although most people will be able to at least attempt the Shoulder Stand (*see pp. 128–31*), it is strongly advised that you don't just "have a go" at this asana before you have first achieved a good level of competence in all the preceding ones. By undertaking the practice in a disciplined fashion you develop, over a period of time, the necessary external and internal strength required to perform these sequences correctly. As with any physically and mentally demanding discipline, it is possible that incorrect practice could lead to injury or disease. Because of the precision required with the earlier asanas, you are strongly advised to learn these postures from a qualified teacher, somebody who has been certified to teach by the Guru, Shri K Pattabhi Jois.

In this phase of the practice session, the foundation and orientation of the body changes from that of the standing and seated asanas. Here, your body will be inverted – thus, your entire weight will be supported on the strength you have developed in your neck and shoulders or, partially, on your head and forearms.

This section of asanas constitutes the climax of the entire practice. The inverted asanas have a powerful effect; they represent the height of purification, and the Shoulder Stand and Head Stand are known as the queen and king of all the asanas. The asanas of the Yoga Chikitsa, or primary series (*see p. 15*), represented by sequences 1 and 2, are designed to mobilize the toxins in the body, while this section of inverted asanas consumes them in the digestive fire (*agni*). The seat of agni is located in the solar plexus, so when the body is inverted the flames, which always travel upward, will cleanse and purify the digestive organs, rectum, and anus.

In order to achieve longevity, people have searched for thousands of years in the hope of discovering some external agent, a magical elixir of life. Yogis, however, discovered long ago that this nectar (known as *amrita bindu*) already existed, but not anywhere in the outside world – they realized that it was located inside their own bodies. The real challenge then became how to preserve and store this internal nectar.

While in a meditative state, the yogis understood that the essence of digested food made blood. The accumulation of 32 droplets of blood is significant because it is this precise amount that is required before blood can be transformed to vitality, or life force. After 32 such transformations have taken place, *amrita bindu* results. The yogis realized that the preservation of *amrita bindu* was a crucial component of life itself, and that without it there is only death.

In our normal upright orientation, the digestive fire acts to consume the droplets of *amrita bindu* in its natural descent from the Sahasrara Chakra, which is the seventh, and highest, energy centre located at the crown of the head. The key to preserving and storing this life-giving nectar is to invert your body, engage the bandhas, and breathe the correct ujjayi breath.

OPPOSITE *Preserving our vital lifeforce,* Salamba Sarvangasana, *the queen of all asanas, purifies the heart, lungs, and all the other parts of the body.*

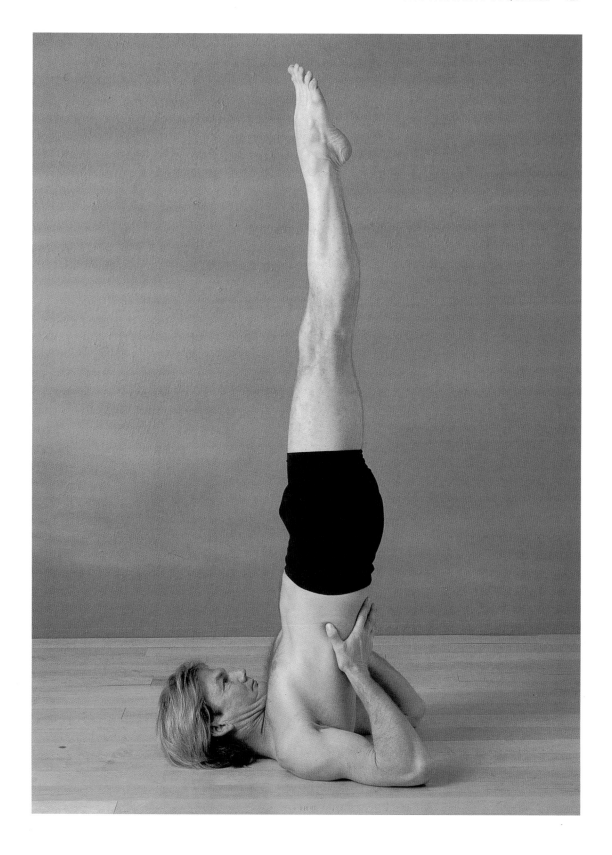

Sequence 3:
Shoulder Stand
Salamba Sarvangasana

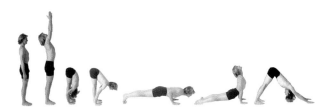

Salamba means "supported" and *Sarvanga*, "all limbs". Traditionally, each shoulder stand and variation has its own full entry and exit vinyasa from *Samasthitih*, but now it is common for the shoulder stand and variations to be combined together as one sequence. In each variation below the traditional vinyasa numbers are used, so the vinyasas shown do not flow from step to step. Each vinyasa follows on from step 2 (vinyasa 7).

It is important to follow the practice rule – start with the *Surya Namaskara*, proceed through the series you are learning, and finish with these asanas. The order is invariable: *Sarvangasana*, *Halasana*, *Karnapidasana*, *Urdhva Padmasana*, *Pindasana*, *Matsyasana*, and finally *Uttanapadasana*.

> **caution**
> Once you have completed these asanas, practise only *Shirhsasana* and *Padmasana*. Performing other asanas after you have completed the finishing asanas is not beneficial.

◀ **1 Vinyasa down**
(Vinyasas 1–6) Flow through this sequence of moves to Downward-facing Dog (*see p. 64*).

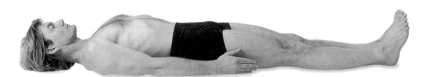

▲ **2 Exhaling (x 5 breaths)**
(Vinyasa 7) From Downward-facing Dog, inhaling, jump through your arms to *Dandasana* and, exhaling, check the line of your spine as you lie down as if in *Samasthitih* (*see p. 110, step 2*). Draw your abdomen in and engage your bandhas. Regulate your breath as you breathe deeply for five steady breaths and look to nasagrai (nose) dristi.

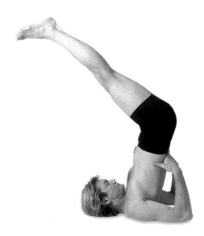

▲ 3 Inhaling

(Vinyasa 8) Roll your arms in to place your hands flat on the mat beside your thighs. Then, using the internal energy harnessed by the bandhas, lift your straight legs off the mat and up into the air. Directing the internal lift up through your legs and, with a push from your arms, raise your buttocks and back off the mat. Now, bending your arms, bring your hands to your waist to support your back.

▶ 4 Inhaling (x 25 breaths)

(Vinyasa 8) Continue to lift your legs, buttocks, and back vertically, up to the point where the entire weight of your body is supported directly on your shoulders. Here, in *Sarvangasana*, you are completely inverted – from your neck to the tips of your toes. Your arms are to be used only as supports; the actual lift must come from your inner body and bandha control. Press your chin into your sternum, gaze to nasagra dristi, and breathe deeply for 25 full breaths.

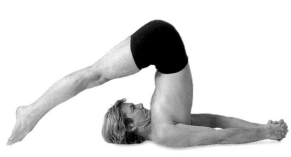

▲ 5 Exhaling (x 10 breaths)

(Vinyasa 8) Exhaling, move to *Halasana*, maintaining bandha control. Keeping the length between your sternum and pubic bone, pivot at your hip and lower your straight legs over your head to the floor. Release your hands from your waist, interlock your fingers behind your back, and straighten your arms, bringing your hands to the floor. Point your toes and pull up on your kneecaps and thighs, keeping your legs active. Continue to focus on nasagrai dristi and breathe deeply for 10 full breaths.

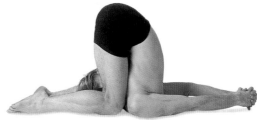

▲ 6 Exhaling (x 10 breaths)

(Vinyasa 8) Exhaling, move to *Karnapidasana*, placing pressure on your ears. Release mula bandha (anus) but keep uddiyana (lower abdomen) engaged. Keep the length between your pubic bone and sternum, and bend your legs. Separate your knees and bring them into contact with the floor and shoulders. Press your knees against your ears and keep your feet together. Gaze to nasagrai dristi and breathe deeply for 10 full breaths. (*For the rest of the sequence turn to next page.*)

▶ **7 Inhaling**

(Vinyasa 8) Return to *Sarvangasana*, unlock your fingers, and, once again, bring your hands to your waist to support your back.

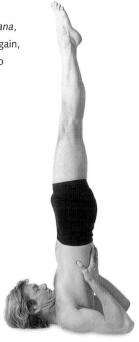

▼ **8 Exhaling**

(Vinyasa 9) Move to *Urdhva Padmasana*. Once again, engage mula bandha and maintain your balance. From *Sarvangasana*, fold your legs down into *Padmasana*. If you can't do this without using your hands, then maintain balance with one hand while you use the other to put your legs, one at a time, into *Padmasana*.

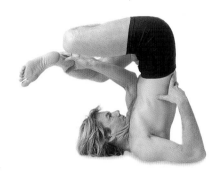

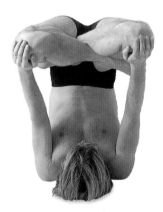

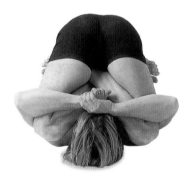

▲ **9 Exhaling (x 10 breaths)**

(Vinyasa 9) While in *Urdhva Padmasana*, inhaling, ensure that your bandha control is present and release the hand support from your back. Maintain your balance and bring your hands to your knees, straighten your arms, and support your *Padmasana*, creating a 90° angle between your legs and back. Engage mula and uddiyana bandhas fully, continue to gaze to nasagrai dristi, and breathe deeply for 10 full breaths.

▲ **10 Exhaling (x 10 breaths)**

(Vinyasa 9) Exhaling, move into *Pindasana*. Release your hands from your knees and slowly bring your *Padmasana* down to rest your knees either side or your head. Wrap your arms around your thighs to bind your *Padmasana*. Hold your fingers or wrists tightly and balance entirely on the back of your head and shoulders. Continue to gaze to nasagrai dristi and breathe deeply for 10 full breaths.

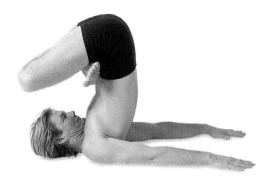

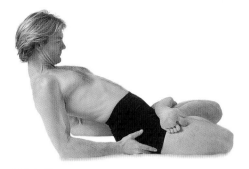

▲ 11 Exhaling

Release your binding and bring your arms once again behind your back, placing your hands on the sides of the mat. Straighten your arms, pressing your palms firmly into the mat. Engage your bandhas, maintaining your head contact with the floor. Now, using the strength of your abdomen and the resistance in your arms, slowly lower your back, one vertebra at a time, down on to the mat.

▲ 12 Exhaling

(Vinyasa 8) Move to *Matsyasana*. Hold the sides of your buttocks, engage your bandhas, and, pressing on your elbows, lift your back off the mat. Roll your pubic bone toward the floor, lengthening through your abdomen, lift your chest, and arch your back. Look to your navel.

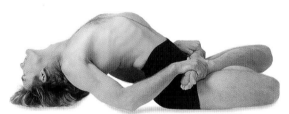

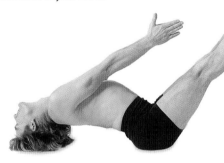

▲ 13 Exhaling (x 10 breaths)

(Vinyasa 8) Continuing to exhale, completely arch your back and place the crown of your head on the mat. Release your hands from your buttocks, lift the pressure from your elbows, and hold your feet. Raise your elbows from the mat and press your knees to the floor. Look to broomadhya (third eye) dristi and breathe deeply for 10 full breaths.

▲ 14 Inhaling (x 10 breaths)

(Vinyasa 8) Move to *Uttanapadasana*. Maintaining the back arch in your upper body, slowly release your legs from *Padmasana*. Without allowing them to touch the floor, straighten and extend them, lifting them as in *Navasana* (see pp. 96–7). Bring the palms of your hands together, straighten your arms, and point your hands to your feet. Look to nasagrai dristi and breathe deeply for 10 full breaths.

▶ 15 Inhaling

While inhaling, bring your hands over your head, placing the palms flat on to the mat with your fingers outstretched and pointing back toward your shoulders, and then perform *Chakrasana*, or Backward Roll (*see pp. 114–15*), landing in *Chatvari* (*see p. 24*).

▼ 16 Vinyasa up

(Vinyasas 11–15) After completing the Backward Roll, flow through this sequence of moves to finish in *Samasthitih* (*see p. 67*).

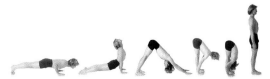

Sequence 3:

Head Stand
Shirhsasana

Shirhsa means "head", and if *Shirhsasana* is executed correctly it is the king of all asanas. Here you stand completely upside down, without any weight on your head, while you support your entire body solely with the strength of your arms, shoulders, and bandhas. Through the correct practice of *Shirhsasana*, the subtle nadis (energy channels) in the brain and sense organs are purified by the increased flow of blood. The vital life-giving nectar, *amrita bindu* (see p. 126), is preserved.

caution
Do not practise this asana if you are pregnant.

◀ **1 Vinyasa down**
(Vinyasas 1–6) Flow through this sequence of moves to Downward-facing Dog (see p. 64).

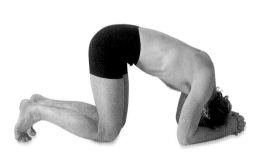

▲ **2 Inhaling**
(Vinyasa 7) From Downward-facing Dog, keep your toes tucked under and sit down on your knees. Bring your elbows down on to the mat, interlock your fingers, and make a triangular-shaped base with your forearms. Bring your shoulders forward over your hands, press through your forearms, and lift out of your shoulder joints. Now, lightly place the crown of your head on the mat and cup the back of your head with your hands.

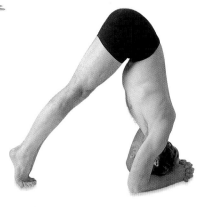

▲ **3 Exhaling**
Pressing strongly through your forearms and elbows, lift from your shoulder joints, and straighten your legs. You may need to walk your toes in toward your face a little so that you can correctly position your buttocks directly above your shoulders. Draw your abdomen in and engage your bandha control. At this point in the sequence you must not collapse your shoulders or place any weight on your head.

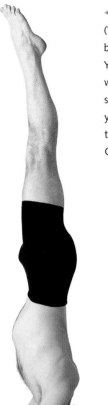

◀ **4 Inhaling (x 25 breaths)**

(Vinyasa 8) Walk your toes in toward your face until your buttocks are positioned a little past the line of your shoulders. Your buttocks will now counterbalance your legs. Continue to work your bandhas, pull up on your kneecaps and thighs, press strongly into the mat with your forearms, and, while inhaling, let your legs float up into the air. When they are vertical, point your toes, draw your lower ribs in, and fully engage your bandhas. Gaze to nasagrai dristi and breathe deeply for 25 full breaths.

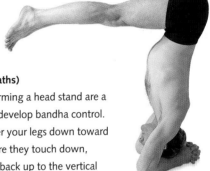

▶ **5 Exhaling (x 5 breaths)**

Leg raises while performing a head stand are a variation designed to develop bandha control. Exhale while you lower your legs down toward the mat, but just before they touch down, inhale and raise them back up to the vertical position. Repeat this five times and then exhale as you position your legs parallel to the floor. Hold this position for five full breaths.

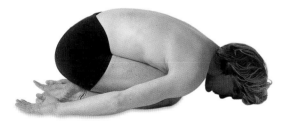

◀ **6 Exhaling–Inhaling**

Exhaling, slowly lower your legs to the floor. Bend your knees, point your feet and sit on your heels. Release your hands, take them back beside your buttocks, and lift and place your forehead on the mat. This is Pose of a Child. Breathe in this position for two minutes.

▶ **7 Vinyasa up**

(Vinyasas 9–13) After completing a two-minute rest in Pose of a Child, flow through this sequence of moves to finish in *Samasthitih* (see p. 67).

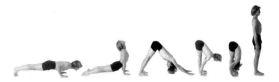

Sequence 3:
Stilling the Waters
Padmasana

Padma translates as "lotus flower". This *Padmasana* sequence, which consists of five variations, is the last of the postures to be woven on to the "thread of the breath". The lotus flower floats on the surface of the water, symbolizing a sense of calm reflection and inner tranquillity. *Yoga Mudra* seals in the energy and stimulates deep cleansing; *Padmasana* regulates the breath, stilling the mind; and *Uth Pluthi* balances the practice.

Follow this final sequence to conclude the Ashtanga Yoga practice: *Baddha Padmasana* (Bound Lotus), *Yoga Mudra* (Final Seal), *Panmasana* (Supported Arch), *Padmasana* (Lotus), and *Uth Pluthi* (Lift).

> **tip**
> *Padmasana* is the classic yoga position for meditation and, apart from their individual benefits, all the other yoga poses are designed to prepare your body to be comfortable in just this one.

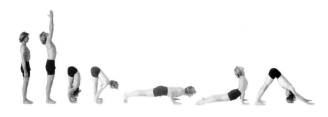

◀ **1 Vinyasa down**
(Vinyasas 1–6) Flow through this sequence of moves to Downward-facing Dog (*see p. 64*).

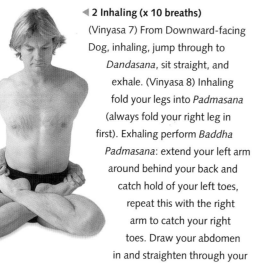

◀ **2 Inhaling (x 10 breaths)**
(Vinyasa 7) From Downward-facing Dog, inhaling, jump through to *Dandasana*, sit straight, and exhale. (Vinyasa 8) Inhaling fold your legs into *Padmasana* (always fold your right leg in first). Exhaling perform *Baddha Padmasana*: extend your left arm around behind your back and catch hold of your left toes, repeat this with the right arm to catch your right toes. Draw your abdomen in and straighten through your spine. Look to nasagrai dristi and breathe deeply for 10 full breaths.

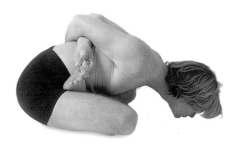

▲ **3 Exhaling (x 10 breaths)**
(Vinyasa 9 – *Yoga Mudra*) Exhaling, press your heels into your lower abdomen and slowly fold your torso over your heels so that your chin comes into contact with the mat. Keep your sit bones in firm contact with the floor. Draw your abdomen in and extend your sternum forward. Look to your broomadhya dristi and breathe deeply for 10 full breaths.

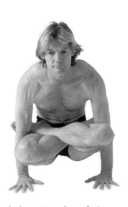

◀ 4 Inhaling (x 10 breaths)

(Vinyasa 10 – *Panmasana*) Inhaling, continue to hold your toes and slowly lift your head and sit upright. Now release your hands and place them on the mat a shoulder-distance apart and approximately 20cm (8in) behind your buttocks. Press your knees, buttocks, and hands into the mat. Arch backward and open your chest. Look to broomadhya dristi and breathe deeply for 10 full breaths.

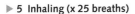

▶ 5 Inhaling (x 25 breaths)

(Vinyasa 8 – *Padmasana*) Inhaling, release your arched back and sit up, bringing your hands to your knees. Join the thumb and index finger of each hand together and straighten your remaining fingers. Draw your abdomen in, lengthen up through your spine without flaring your ribs, and tuck your chin gently down into your sternum. Look to nasagrai dristi and breathe deeply for 25 full breaths.

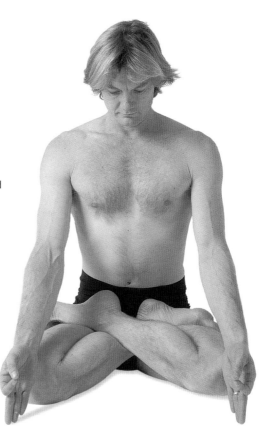

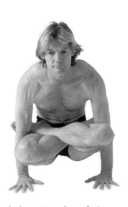

▲ 6 Inhaling (x 25 breaths)

(Vinyasa 9 – *Uth Pluthi*) Exhaling, place your hands on the mat beside your thighs and engage your bandhas. Lift your knees up toward your chest, press through your palms, and, inhaling, lift your body right off the mat. Straighten your arms, look to nasagrai dristi, and breathe deeply for 25 full breaths.

▼ 7 Vinyasa up

(Vinyasas 10–14) Flow through this sequence of moves to finish in *Samasthitih* (see p. 67). Now lie down, cover yourself with a blanket, and rest.

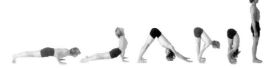

CLOSING MANTRA

Om
Swasthi-praja bhyah pari pala yantam
Nya-yena margena mahi-mahishaha
Go-bramanebhyaha-shuhamastu-nityam
Lokaa-samastha sukhino-bhavanthu
Om

Om
May prosperity be glorified
May administrators rule the world with law and justice
May all things that are sacred be protected
And may people of the world be happy and prosperous
Om

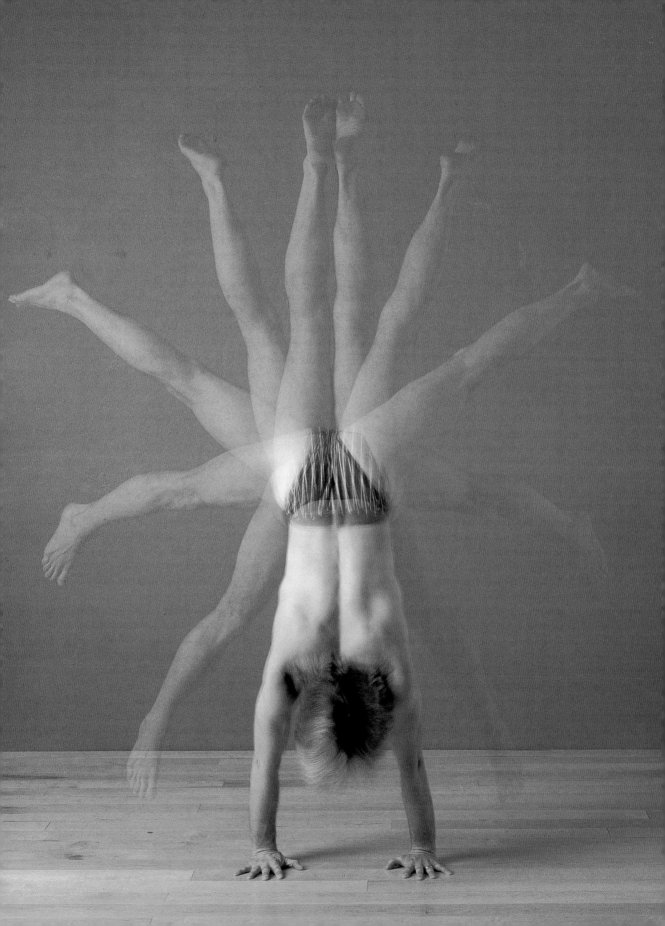

RESOURCES

If you are interested in furthering your study of Ashtanga Yoga, you should make contact with any of the following individuals or institutions.

AUSTRALIA

Eileen Hall
Yoga Moves
The Verona Building
17 Oxford Street
Paddington
NSW 2021

Dena Kingsberg
PO Box 1443
Byron Bay
NSW 2481

Graeme & Leonie
Northfield
PO Box 220
Cooroy
Queensland 4563

FINLAND

Stefan Engstrom
The Midnight Sun Ashtanga
Yoga Retreat
Sando Strom
10900 Hanko

FRANCE

Odile Morcrette
20 Rue Fenelon
59000 Lille

Philippe Mons
86 Rue De La Gare
59350 St Andre

Brigitte De Rose
74 Boulevard Gambetta
62100 Calais

GREECE

Radha & Pierre
Yoga Plus
Agios Pavlos
Crete

INDIA

Shri K Pattabhi Jois
Ashtanga Yoga Nilayam
876/1 1st Cross
Laxmipuram
Mysore 570004

ITALY

Lino Miele & Tina Pizzimenti
Ashatanga Yoga School
Via Cassia 698
00189 Rome

NEW ZEALAND

Gwendoline Hunt
17 Creswick Terrace
Wellington

Peter Nielson & Jude Hynes
Auckland Yoga Academy
1st Floor 33 High Street
Central City
Auckland

Andre Moffat
The Ashtanga Room
18 Eden Street
Newmarket
Auckland

SPAIN

Tomas Zorzo & Camino Diez
Astanga Yoga Center
C/ San Bernabe 7 ñ3a
33002 Oviedo

SWEDEN

Maria Boox
Sodermalms Yogashala
Gotlandsgatan 86
11631 Stockholm

Gitan Hendele
Ashtanga Stockholm
Gammelgard SV 34
11264 Stockholm

UNITED KINGDOM

Hamish Hendry
Yoga Therapy Cenre
60 Great Ormond Street
London WC1N

Kristina Karitinos Ireland
c/o Natural Health Centre
27 Regent Street
Brighton BN1 1UL

Gingi Lee
Sangam Yoga Centre
80a Battersea Rise
London SW11 1EH

John Scott & Lucy Scott
The Space at No8
8 Chapel Street
Penzance TR18 4AJ

TRI YOGA
Unit 4
6 Erskine Road
Primrose Hill
London NW3

The Yoga Centre
1 Meadow Place
Edinburgh EH9 1JZ

UNITED STATES OF
AMERICA

Richard Freeman
The Yoga Workshop
2020 21st Street
Boulder
CO 80302

Sharon Gannon & David Life
Jivamukti Yoga Center
404 Lafayette Street
3rd Floor
New York
NY 10003

Chuck Miller & Maty Ezraty
Yoga Works
2215 Main Street

Santa Monica
CA 90405

Tim Miller
Ashtanga Yoga Center
118 West E Street
Encinitas
CA 90049

Annie Pace
PO BOX 125
Crestone
CO 81131

Eddie & Jocelyn Stern
Patanjali Yoga Shala
611 Broadway Suite 203
New York
NY 10012

FURTHER READING

Highly recommended
Jois, Shri K Pattabhi, *Yoga Mala*, Patanjali Yoga Shala, NewYork, 2000

Miele, Lino, *Astanga Yoga*, Lino Miele, Rome, 1999

Swenson, David, *Ashtanga Yoga The Practice Manual*, Ashtanga Yoga Productions, Texas, 1999

General interest
Desikachar, TKV (with Cravens, RH), *Yoga and the Living Tradition of Krishnamacharya*, Aperture Foundation, Hong Kong, 1998

Feurstein, Georg, *The Yoga Tradition, Its History, Literature, Philosophy and Practice*, Hohm Press, Arizona, 1998

Saraswati, Swami Sayananda, *Moola Bandha, The Master Key*, Bihar School of Yoga, Bihar, 1996

Satchidananda, Sri Swami (translation and commentary), *The Yoga Sutras of Pantanjali*, Integral Yoga Publications, Virginia, 1997

Schiffmann, Erich, *Yoga, The Spirit and Practice of Moving into Stillness*, Pocket Books, USA, 1996

Sjoman, NE, *Yoga Tradition of the Mysore Palace*, Abhinav Publications, New Delhi, 1996

INDEX

ACKNOWLEDGEMENTS

I would like to thank the following people for their support and encouragement in the production of this book.

First and foremost thanks go to my dearly loved wife, Lucy Scott, for her additional knowledge, writing skills, love, support, and encouragement. Also to Shri K Pattabhi Jois for all his wisdom and his willingness to share it, and his untiring dedication to the teaching and the preservation of Ashtanga Yoga, without which my life work would not exist. To know Guruji enriches my spirit beyond words.

Thanks to Sharath, for his years of dedication to the practice and teaching of Ashtanga Yoga, for all those adjustments and for being an inspiration to me. And to Derek Ireland, for being my first teacher, and so much more.

To Hamish Hendry, for his love, friendship, honest opinions, and for the translation of the Sanskrit titles. Also, on my behalf, thanks for presenting the first draft of this book by hand to Guruji.

My thanks go to Eddie Stern, for his friendship, love, wisdom, guidance, and always having the time when help is needed. My appreciation, too, for supplying the photograph of Guruji. To Gingi Lee, for his love, friendship and kindness, and for allowing us to photograph a class in action at the Sangam Yoga Centre.

To Kristina Karitinos-Ireland, for her strength, love, and the continuation of Derek's work, and her generosity in supplying the photograph of Derek Ireland. To Tom Sewall, for capturing such a characteristic image of Guruji and for allowing me to use the photograph. Thanks to Joseph Dunham, for his time and wisdom and for acting as my political advisor. And to Tony Rutland, for his kind heart, generosity, time, and patience, and also for his integrity and for sharing his legal knowledge with me.

I would also like to express my appreciation to all the students, for providing the opportunity for me to explore the method and the practice, and thus teaching me so much.

My thanks also go to the photographic models, Lucy Scott, Bumni Daramola, Paula Bennett, and the students of the Sangam Yoga Centre, and of course to photographers Paul Forrester and Colin Bowling for their diligence, patience, attention to detail, and their sense of fun during the photographic sessions.

And my special thanks go to both my editor Jonathan Hilton and graphic designer Peggy Sadler for their willingness to learn and their unrelenting patience. Also for their flexibility in allowing me such freedom in the presentation.

Gaia Books would like to thank Susanna Abbott for proofreading and Lynn Bresler for indexing.

Photograph on page 11: *Shiva* (AKG London/Jean-Louis Nou, Jaipur, Collection Sangaram Singh).